BARIATRIC PLASTIC SURGERY

A Guide to Cosmetic Surgery after Weight Loss

THOMAS B. MCNEMAR, M.D. • JOHN LOMONACO, M.D. • MITCHEL D. KRIEGER, M.D.

Addicus Books, Inc.
Omaha, Nebraska

An Addicus Nonfiction Book

ISBN 978-1-886039-92-6

Cover design by Janice St. Marie

Typography by Linda Dageforde

Illustrations by Jack Kusler

This book is not intended to serve as a substitute for a physician. Nor is it the authors' intent to give medical advice contrary to that of an attending physician.

Library of Congress Cataloging-in-Publication Data

McNemar, Thomas, 1962-
    Bariatric plastic surgery : a guide to cosmetic surgery after weight loss / Thomas B. McNemar, Mitchel D. Krieger, John LoMonaco.
       p. cm.
"An Addicus nonfiction book."
Includes index.
ISBN 978-1-886039-92-6 (alk. paper)
1. Obesity—Surgery. 2. Surgery, Plastic. 3. Weight loss. I. Krieger, Mitchel D., 1962- II. LoMonaco, John, 1963- III. Title.
RD540.M4257 2008
617.4'3—dc22   2008024785

Addicus Books, Inc.
P.O. Box 45327
Omaha, Nebraska 68145
www.AddicusBooks.com

Printed in the United States of America
10 9 8 7 6 5 4 3 2 1

To my wife, Cindy, and my children, Mackenzie and Kelsey.
May you always follow your dreams.
—Thomas B. McNemar, M.D., F.A.C.S.

To my family for their understanding and support, especially during my
long absences. To my father John LoMonaco Sr., whose indomitable
spirit exemplifies perseverance and drive.
—John LoMonaco, M.D., F.A.C.S.

To my wife, Colleen, for your love, support, and understanding.
To my father, Jerry Krieger, for your love and for the example you have set for me.
You have provided me a moral compass with which to guide my life.
To the memory of my mother, Barbara Krieger, who ignited my love for medicine,
and whose courage and tenacity remain an inspiration to me.
—Mitchel D. Krieger, M.D., F.A.C.S.

Contents

Acknowledgments

A book of this type requires many different talents. I would like to thank Rod Colvin and Frances Sharpe for bringing the book together. I thank my two colleagues, Dr. Krieger and Dr. LoMonaco, for their insights, and I acknowledge my staff, Danielle Hall and Tiffany Pederson. I would like to thank all my patients, past and future. I also thank my family, Cindy, Mackenzie, and Kelsey. I am blessed to have them.

Thomas D. McNemar, M.D., F.A.C.S.

This book would not have been possible without the concerted efforts of my colleagues and the dedication of all my staff. It is our patients, however, who have inspired us. To them we owe the greatest thanks. Their confidence in our abilities is the reason we are here.

John LoMonaco, M.D., F.A.C.S.

The support of many individuals have made this book possible. First, I would like to thank my wonderful and talented wife, Col. Colleen Shull. Your enthusiasm and love for your soldiers is truly inspirational. Our country is fortunate to have someone so talented to lead our troops and provide an example for those around her. I also would like to thank my family for their encouragement and unconditional love. I've journeyed down many paths throughout my career, always returning home to find their support and love unwavering.

I also would like to thank my staff for their dedication and efforts to provide the finest care possible for our patients. Each day is a collaborative effort, and I am truly grateful for their contributions. I wish to thank Frances Sharpe for her editorial support and for our many enjoyable conversations. Finally, I would like to thank my patients, who never cease to amaze me. Your remarkable capacity to support and love those around you is astounding. I thank you all for bringing me into your community knowing that the relationships I have developed with you will last a lifetime.

Mitchel D. Krieger, M.D., F.A.C.S.

Introduction

Congratulations! You've succeeded in losing a great deal of weight. This is no easy task, and you should be proud of your achievement. Whether you've lost weight thanks to a bariatric procedure or you've done it the old-fashioned way with diet and exercise, it takes a strong commitment and a healthy dose of willpower. By shedding those extra pounds, you've probably noted countless changes for the better in your health and in your daily life. For instance, you may have experienced improvements in your blood pressure or with diabetes, two health problems commonly associated with being overweight. You also may have significantly increased your physical stamina and your ability to enjoy an active life. Now that you've reached or are nearing your weight goal, you deserve to feel good about yourself and your new shape.

Unfortunately, losing large amounts of weight can sometimes create other troublesome body issues. In particular, loose and excess skin may prevent you from fully enjoying the results of your weight loss efforts.

Excess skin that hangs from your body can cause skin irritations and rashes. In addition, loose, hanging skin can keep you from seeing your body's true new size and can force you to continue wearing larger sizes of clothing. A visible reminder of the weight you used to carry, excess skin may even leave you feeling a bit blue.

Take heart that you are not alone. Excess skin affects many men and women who have lost large amounts of weight. The good news is that there are a number of plastic surgery procedures that address the problem of loose skin after weight loss. In fact, the demand for such procedures has grown dramatically in the past few years. And plastic surgeons have answered the call with refinements in techniques and innovative procedures that can help you achieve a more pleasing shape.

This book is designed to help you understand the various procedures available and to answer some of your questions about what to expect from plastic surgery after weight loss. From choosing a surgeon to recovering from surgery at home, *Bariatric Plastic Surgery: A Guide to Cosmetic Surgery after Weight Loss* will help guide you on your journey to an improved body shape, better health, and an enhanced quality of life.

Contemplating Bariatric Plastic Surgery

If you've spent years battling excess fat, you should feel very proud of yourself for losing a large amount of weight. But shedding all those pounds may not have given you the body contours you desire. In fact, your massive weight loss may have caused a new problem you hadn't anticipated, namely, excess skin that hangs in folds on your body. This sagging skin may be preventing you from seeing your slimmer new shape and may actually make you feel disappointed with your new look. You may feel that the loose skin is an unpleasant reminder of your former self or that you still feel overweight when you look in the mirror.

Loose skin also may be causing hygiene and health problems and may be making it hard for you to find clothing that fits. And unfortunately, no amount of dieting or exercise is going to eliminate all that extra skin or make it shrink to fit your new shape. Plastic surgery can add an important psycho-logical benefit to the health benefits you have already received from your weight loss.

Considering all the effort you put into losing weight, all this loose skin can be extremely frustrating. Fortunately, there are several cosmetic surgery procedures that can remove excess skin and give you the sleeker body you've worked so hard to achieve.

What Is Bariatric Plastic Surgery after Weight Loss?

Plastic surgery after weight loss is designed to enhance the shape of your body. It aims to improve the proportions of your figure and to improve your skin tone by removing the loose, sagging skin that often follows massive weight loss. Some of these surgical procedures also tighten underlying tissues or remove fat deposits to produce a more aesthetically pleasing shape. Cosmetic surgery can address the problem of loose skin on nearly every part of your body as well as on your face and neck.

Types of Bariatric Plastic Surgery

Several different surgical procedures are available to improve your body contours. Commonly performed procedures are designed to target sagging skin on the abdomen, thighs, buttocks, breasts, chest, back, arms, face, and neck. Following is a list of plastic surgery procedures that can be performed following weight loss to give you a more pleasing shape.

- *Tummy Tuck:* Also called *abdominoplasty,* a tummy tuck is a surgical procedure that resculpts the shape of your abdomen. It can give you a smoother, flatter-looking belly and a more well-defined waistline. The procedure removes excess skin from the abdomen, and it also can tighten underlying tissues and remove stubborn fat that hasn't responded to your weight loss efforts. The belly button also is reconstructed, and rejuvenation of the pubic area is frequently performed.

- *Panniculectomy:* This surgical procedure is designed specifically to remove a *panniculus*—also referred to as a *pannus*—a large apron of skin and fat that hangs from the abdomen and is a fairly common occurrence following massive weight loss. The goal of a panniculectomy often is to remove massive amounts of skin and fat that may be causing infection or serious limitations in your activity. A panniculectomy typically does not have the same aesthetic outcome as a tummy tuck but can still help redefine the shape of your abdomen.

- *Thigh Lift:* Also called *thighplasty,* a thigh lift can eliminate drooping skin from the inner and/or outer thighs to give you more shapely legs. By tightening the remaining skin, thigh lift surgery may rid you of unsightly saddlebags and, in some cases, also may reduce the appearance of cellulite.

- *Buttocks Lift:* This surgical procedure improves the shape of your posterior by getting rid of sagging skin and restoring skin tone.

- *Pubic Lift:* A pubic lift, also called *monsplasty,* can alleviate the severe sagging and bulky tissue buildup in the pubic area that sometimes accompanies massive weight loss.

- *Body Lift:* Also referred to as a *lower body lift, belt lipectomy, central body lift,* or *circumferential torsoplasty,* a body lift improves the contours of the abdomen, thighs, and buttocks. This surgical procedure typically combines a tummy

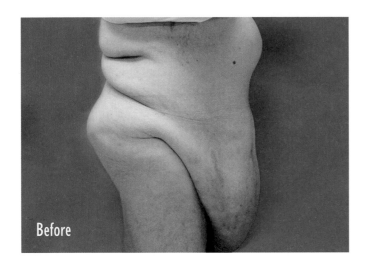

Before

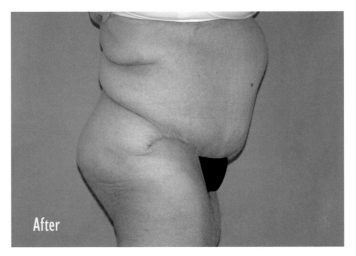

After

The apron of loose skin hanging from the abdomen is called a panniculus. This patient underwent a panniculectomy, a procedure performed to remove the panniculus for both cosmetic and functional purposes.

tuck, pubic lift *(monsplasty),* thigh lift, and buttocks lift into a single operation.

- *Breast Lift:* With a breast lift, also called *mastopexy,* droopy breasts are restored to a more pleasing and youthful shape. With breast lift surgery, excess skin is removed, and the remaining, tightened skin provides better support to the breast tissue. In some cases, breast implants may be used to help fill out the shape of breasts that have deflated after weight loss. This is called a *breast lift with augmentation.*

- *Breast Reduction:* With breast reduction surgery, breasts that are too large following weight loss can be reduced to a size that is in better proportion with the new contours of your body.

- *Male Breast Reduction:* This surgical procedure aims to restore a more natural shape to the male chest by eliminating the breast enlargement that can result from being overweight.

- *Arm Lift:* Also called *brachioplasty,* an arm lift is a surgical procedure that can eliminate skin that hangs down from the back of your arms.

- *Upper Body Lift:* This surgical procedure is designed to improve the contours of the breasts (or the male chest), upper back, and arms. An upper body lift typically combines a number of procedures into the same operation.

- *Facelift:* With a facelift, also called *rhytidectomy,* you can achieve a more youthful, rested look. A facelift tightens the jowls as well as the underlying muscles to enhance your appearance.

- *Neck Lift:* Often performed at the same time as a facelift, a neck lift, also called *cervicoplasty,* provides greater definition to the jawline and neck by removing loose skin.

- *Liposuction:* One of the most popular of all cosmetic surgical procedures, liposuction is used to permanently remove fat from a variety of areas of the body. It is commonly used in conjunction with other bariatric plastic surgery procedures to help you achieve the sleeker contours you want.

Growing Popularity of Plastic Surgery after Weight Loss

The popularity of plastic surgery after weight loss is escalating rapidly. This rise is directly related to the increase in the number of Americans who are undergoing some form of bariatric surgery to accelerate weight loss. Bariatric surgery involves a number of procedures performed on the stomach and/or intestines either to restrict food intake or to alter the way food is processed and absorbed. The typical result is rapid weight loss.

Currently, each year, more than 200,000 Americans have some form of bariatric surgery to accelerate weight loss. And that number is climbing quickly. With the rapid weight loss experienced following bariatric surgery, sagging skin is an unfortunate by-product. That's why more than 55,000 men and women who have undergone bariatric surgery seek out some form of cosmetic surgery following weight loss.

Of course, having bariatric surgery isn't the only way to lose large amounts of weight, and it isn't the only reason that cosmetic surgery following weight loss is surging in popularity. If you shed pounds the old-fashioned way with diet and exercise, you can still be saddled with excess flesh, which can motivate you to seek a surgical solution. Rest assured that the plastic surgery procedures covered in this book are designed to improve your body contours regardless of how you lost weight.

Are You a Candidate for Bariatric Plastic Surgery?

If you've dropped a significant amount of weight and are now bothered by drooping skin, you may be a candidate for plastic surgery. The various procedures available can be tailored for women or men and are usually highly individualized to meet your specific needs. Provided you're in good overall health, dramatic improvements can be achieved whether you're in your twenties or in your golden years.

Plastic surgeons will look at several factors to determine if you are a good candidate for surgery. These factors include your weight, your overall health, your age, your expectations, and your attitude.

Your Weight

One of the key factors surgeons look at when deciding if you would make a good candidate for post–weight loss plastic surgery is your weight. More important than the actual number, however, is how long your weight has been stable. Stable means that your weight fluctuates no more than a few pounds. Most physicians recommend waiting to have surgery until your weight has been stable for approximately three to six months or more. With a stable weight, you are more likely to achieve the best results from surgery.

Some surgeons also take your body mass index (BMI) into consideration. Your BMI is the ratio between your weight and your height and is a good indicator of whether you are normal, overweight, obese, or morbidly obese. A BMI of 18 to 24 is associated with normal weight, 25 to 29 indicates you are overweight, 30 to 39 puts you in the obese category, and 40 or more suggests morbid obesity.

In general, the lower your BMI, the better your results will be. Ideally, your BMI should be below 30 in order to ensure the best possible outcome. You may still be considered a candidate for surgery if your BMI is in the 30 to 35 range or even slightly higher. In this range, however, you should be aware that the risk for complications increases and that the results typically aren't as satisfactory.

Your Overall Health

Your overall health is one of the most important things plastic surgeons take into consideration when determining if you're a candidate for surgery. Fortunately, your health may have improved significantly since losing weight. In many cases, shedding pounds can lessen or completely alleviate many medical conditions that are associated with obesity, such as type 2 diabetes, hypertension, sleep apnea, and heart disease.

Your Age

You don't have to fall within a specific age range to have plastic surgery following weight loss. However, if you are older, your overall health condition may be of more concern. Anyone over the age of forty may be required to obtain medical clearance from your physician before surgery. Being sixty or beyond also may play a role in determining which procedures are most appropriate for you and whether or not you can have more than one procedure performed during the same operation.

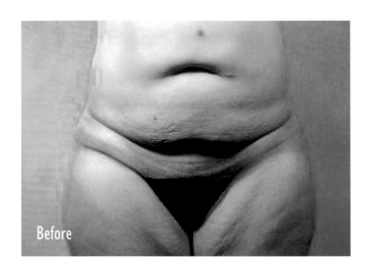

Before

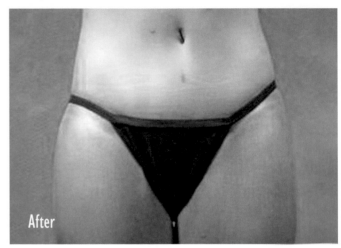

After

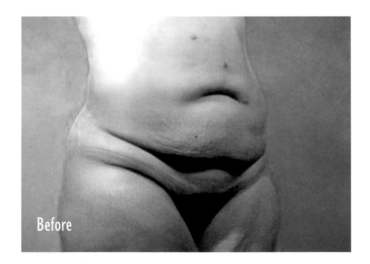

Before

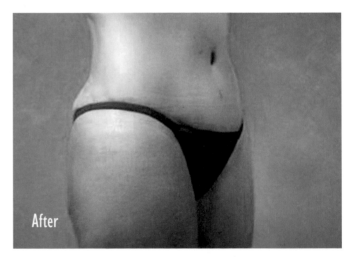

After

Lower body lift with inner and outer thigh lift

Your Expectations

Having realistic expectations is one of the most important qualifications if you're considering plastic surgery after weight loss. Plastic surgeons stress that the key word you need to focus on is "improvement" rather than "perfection." This is true regardless of which post–weight loss procedure or procedures interest you the most. If you're willing to accept this fact, you'll be a better candidate for surgery. In addition, you'll have a much higher chance of being satisfied with your results.

You also need to anticipate a significant amount of scarring as a result of surgical procedures that remove excess skin. These scars may appear on several parts of your body depending on the procedures performed. It's important that you fully understand that these scars can be quite extensive. Fortunately, in many cases, the scars can be placed strategically so they will be hidden from view by your clothing or even by a bathing suit. If you're like most people who opt for plastic surgery, scars are a very acceptable trade-off for a better body contour.

Be aware, too, that the recovery period following plastic surgery after weight loss can be rather lengthy. In fact, it can take quite a bit longer to recover from post–weight loss surgery than it does to bounce back from bariatric surgery itself. Depending on the specific surgical procedures you have, you may be required to spend a day or two in the hospital, and your recovery may take several weeks or even more than a month. Because of this, you should be prepared to miss work for some period of time after having your procedure.

Your Attitude

Having a healthy attitude is another desirable factor in candidates for plastic surgery after weight loss. It's best if you're emotionally stable and have a positive attitude about yourself. Of course, living with unsightly, droopy skin can wreak havoc with your self-esteem and self-confidence. It's understandable that you might have some lingering negative feelings about the way your body looks. These feelings can often be alleviated once surgery removes that extra baggage. However, if you harbor negative feelings about yourself in general, your new look may not remedy these feelings.

A good attitude also means being willing to take an active role in the experience. This involves taking the time to learn about the various procedures that might be right for you, asking questions, communicating your goals clearly, and following instructions carefully. By being an active participant in the surgery process, you greatly increase your chances of achieving optimal results.

Understanding the Limitations of Plastic Surgery after Weight Loss

Good candidates realize that even though plastic surgery procedures can reshape your body to give it more pleasing contours, there are physical limitations to what can be achieved. For instance, no amount of surgery can alter your basic bone structure. If your hip bones are wide or if your rib cage is asymmetrical, removing excess skin won't change that and may in fact make it more noticeable. Also, it's important to note that the more loose flesh you have, the harder it is to obtain optimal results.

Remember that these procedures are designed mainly to eliminate and tighten loose skin; they aren't considered a treatment for obesity, cellulite, or stretch marks. Yes, some fat can be removed along with your excess skin, but plastic surgery shouldn't be viewed as a weight loss method. Tightening the skin and removing fat deposits may reduce the appearance of cellulite in some cases but can't be expected to make it disappear. And only stretch marks that are located within the areas of skin to be removed will be eliminated.

When Bariatric Plastic Surgery Is Not Recommended

Having plastic surgery following massive weight loss isn't right for everybody. For example, if you suffer from certain medical conditions, plastic surgery may not be suitable for you. Health problems that may prevent you from being considered a good candidate for surgery include:

- Heart disease
- Lung disease
- Kidney disease
- Liver disease
- Uncontrolled diabetes
- Uncontrolled hypertension
- Bleeding disorders
- Connective-tissue diseases
- Endocrine diseases
- Autoimmune diseases

If you are still severely obese, you may not be considered a good candidate. In this case, a plastic surgeon may recommend that you postpone surgery until you are closer to your goal weight. Likewise, if you hope to continue losing weight, it may be best to wait until you've reached a weight you would like to maintain.

In general, smokers do not make good candidates for post–weight loss procedures. That's because nicotine—whether it's delivered via cigarettes, gum, the patch, or chewing tobacco—can diminish the body's ability to heal wounds after surgery. And because the incisions for these procedures are extensive, proper wound healing is critical to a successful outcome.

Having unrealistic expectations usually indicates that you aren't an ideal candidate for surgery. That's because even if you achieve the best possible results, you probably still won't be happy with your outcome.

Timing of Your Surgery: How Soon after Weight Loss?

Even though you may be eager to have cosmetic surgery to complement your weight loss and to complete your new look, it's best to wait for some time after shedding those extra pounds. Depending on your surgeon, you may be asked to delay surgery until you've stabilized your weight for three to six months or even longer.

If you've had some form of bariatric surgery, it usually takes approximately twelve to eighteen months before you are ready to be evaluated for cosmetic procedures. However, some people lose weight more slowly than others, and it may take longer. For instance, some types of bariatric surgery, such as lap band surgery, produce a more gradual weight loss. In this case, it may take two to three years before you are ready for plastic surgery.

Having a stable weight is key for several reasons. If you are still in the process of losing weight rapidly, your *metabolism* may be altered. This may limit your body's ability to heal wounds following major surgery. In addition, it may lead to a depressed immune system, leaving you more vulnerable to infection. Usually, your body's immune system and wound healing capabilities return to full force once your weight has stabilized.

For instance, you may experience nausea and vomiting during the first few months after bariatric surgery. This can lead to an imbalance in your *electrolytes*, the minerals in blood that regulate the amount of fluid in your body. Low levels of electrolytes can put you at increased risk for complications as a result of anesthesia. With time, proper nutrition, and dietary counseling, your body will adjust to the changes in your digestive system, and you should be able to keep your electrolytes balanced.

In addition, it's important to give your skin a chance to contract naturally to your new shape. Even though many people who shed significant girth will not experience any tightening of the skin, some individuals will notice some degree of retraction. And typically, the less extra skin you have, the better the results you can achieve from surgery.

Multiple Procedures

If you have skin hanging from more than one area of your body, you'll probably need multiple procedures to reach your goals. For instance, if your skin is saggy on your abdomen, you may benefit from a tummy tuck, but this may not be enough to give you the look you desire. You also may benefit from a thigh lift, a buttocks lift, or some other procedure. In fact, it's very common to need several procedures to achieve the best outcome. This can be accomplished either by combining procedures into a single operation or by staging procedures in a series of operations.

Combining Procedures

When multiple procedures are required, your plastic surgeon may recommend combining procedures into a single operation. For instance, your surgeon may suggest having a tummy tuck, thigh lift, and buttocks lift all on the same day, or an arm lift and a breast lift in one operation. Combining procedures offers several advantages. For example, by having multiple procedures performed at the same time, you reduce your exposure to anesthesia, and you face only one recovery period and one period of time off work. In addition, the results following surgery are likely to be far more dramatic.

However, combining procedures poses drawbacks, too. For instance, it may raise your risk for complications both during your procedure and after you return home to recover. In addition, it lengthens your recovery period and may make you more uncomfortable as you heal. The surgeon's choice of a well-equipped facility to manage the early phases of your recovery and to respond effectively to your needs is most important, especially when considering the more extensive combined procedures.

As you can imagine, any surgical procedure can cause some soreness and can reduce your ability to move around in the days following your operation. For example, if you have a thigh lift, post-operative soreness in your legs might make it difficult to walk around, to get out of bed, or to sit down. In this instance, you would probably rely more heavily on your arms to help you get up and down. But if you've had an arm lift in the same operation, you might not be able to do so, and your mobility would be further restricted. Since movement is one of the keys to a healthy recovery, an increased lack of mobility puts you more at risk for developing complications.

In addition, there are limits to the number of procedures that can safely be performed during a single operation. In general, most surgeons recommend limiting the amount of time you're in surgery to approximately six to eight hours. Beyond this limit, the risks associated with surgery and the exposure to anesthesia increase.

However, some physicians do perform a total body lift that combines a lower body lift and an upper body lift in the same operation. Typically, this type of procedure is performed with a team of two or three surgeons and takes about ten to twelve hours to complete. Although the total body lift can produce dramatic results, it also requires an extensive recovery period and increases the risk of complications both during and after the surgery. For these reasons, most plastic surgery specialists do not advocate having a total body lift.

Staging Procedures

To ensure your safety, your surgeon may recommend staging your procedures. This means that you will have a series of operations spaced out over a period of time. For many post–weight loss patients, it's common to have two or three operations to complete the process. Depending on how many areas of your body are affected by excess skin, you may need as many as five operations to achieve the results you want.

After each operation, your body needs ample time to heal before you can safely have another procedure. The exact length of time depends on how your individual recovery goes, but most surgeons recommend waiting approximately two to six months before having subsequent procedures. Therefore, it can take a year or two—or even more in some cases—to complete the process. When contemplating this time, remember that it likely took many years for your skin to reach the condition it is in, so be patient, and allow your surgeon several sessions to correct everything safely. The old saying "Rome wasn't built in a day" certainly applies here.

Staging procedures doesn't mean, however, that you are only having one single procedure with each operation. For example, you may have a combined tummy tuck, thigh lift, and buttocks lift in one operation and then a breast lift and an arm lift in a subsequent operation. Since every individual is unique, there is no blueprint for staging procedures. Depending on your body and your goals, your surgeon will determine the best and safest combination of procedures and staging of operations for you.

Your safety is the main benefit of staging procedures. In addition, the recovery period following staged procedures is likely to be quicker than if you have an all-in-one total body lift. Staging procedures also may lead to a better overall outcome because it allows your surgeon to fine-tune your results in the following operations. For instance, let's say you have a lower body lift for your first operation and an upper body lift for your second operation. During your second operation, your surgeon can make minor improvements to your abdomen, thighs, or buttocks if necessary.

The disadvantages of staging procedures are that you will be exposed to anesthesia with each operation, and you will have more than one recovery period. In spite of this, the vast majority of plastic surgeons recommend staging as the best and safest way to accomplish your goals.

What's the Next Step?

Only a plastic surgeon can determine if you are indeed a good candidate for surgery after weight loss and which procedures will best help you achieve your goals, so schedule an appointment for a consultation. Prior to your meeting, spend some time learning about the various procedures that interest you. Meet with other patients who have had the procedures, or read about their experiences. Your surgeon's office will likely have many of these important resources available for you. This way, you'll be prepared to ask questions about the surgery process and to communicate your goals effectively.

2

Choosing a Plastic Surgeon

One of the most important decisions you'll make regarding plastic surgery after weight loss is choosing your surgeon. Thousands of plastic surgeons nationwide perform the procedures that can help you achieve more flattering body contours, but how do you know which one is right for you? Knowing what to look for in terms of training and experience can help you narrow your choices. But those aren't the only qualifications that count. Finding a surgeon with whom you feel comfortable is also key. When you feel at ease with your surgeon, you are more likely to have good communication, which often increases your chances of having satisfactory results. Because your choice of surgeon is so critical to your overall outcome, you should be prepared to spend some quality time on this crucial step.

Finding a Plastic Surgeon

You have many options when it comes to finding a qualified plastic surgeon. A good first step is to ask your friends, family, and physicians for referrals. If you belong to a support group for weight loss patients, consider asking the members of your group for recommendations. Likewise, if you had bariatric surgery, check with the doctor who performed your procedure. Many bariatric specialists maintain professional relationships with local area plastic surgeons and routinely offer referrals. Once you have a list of names, visit each doctor's Web site. This can give you a better idea about the surgeon's practice and experience with post–weight loss plastic surgery procedures.

You also can use the Internet to search for physicians. But be aware that not all plastic surgery Web sites are the same. Many sites are

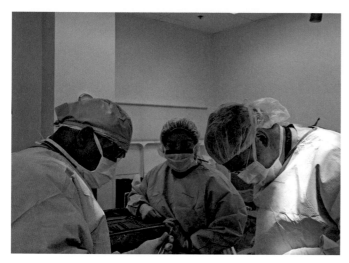

Choosing an experienced, board-certified plastic surgeon is the first step in ensuring good results with bariatric plastic surgery.

simply commercial for-profit ventures that will list any plastic surgeon for a fee without verifying qualifications, training, or experience. When searching for a plastic surgery specialist, you may want to confine your Internet search to reputable medical organizations, such as the American Society of Plastic Surgeons (www.plasticsurgery.org). This site offers a handy physician-finder tool to help you locate qualified surgeons in your area.

Surgeon Qualifications: What to Look For

Of course, you want to choose a surgeon who is highly qualified. But what exactly makes a surgeon qualified? In general, any surgeon you're considering should have the proper education and training, should be board certified, and should have experience performing bariatric plastic surgery procedures.

Education and Training

Several years of formal education and specialized training are required to become a plastic surgeon. The first step in the lengthy process is graduating from a four-year college or university, followed by the successful completion of an additional four years at medical school. The medical school should be *accredited,* which means that the institution meets standards set by a national authority for medical education programs.

After earning an M.D. degree from medical school, doctors who want to become plastic surgeons must complete several years of additional hands-on training. This training begins with at least five years of hospital training called a residency. During the residency, doctors perform surgery under the guidance of senior-level surgeons. The first few years of the residency typically cover general surgery procedures. The focus shifts to plastic surgery procedures during the last few years of the residency. Doctors take on increasing amounts of responsibility as their residency progresses. By the time they complete the residency, they've gained ample hands-on surgical experience and are able to assume responsibility for the complete care of patients.

After the residency is completed, many plastic surgeons choose to continue their training with a fellowship that concentrates on a specialized area of plastic surgery. However, training doesn't end there. In order to maintain certification, all plastic surgeons are required to take continuing medical education courses as long as they remain in practice. This provides assurance that doctors remain up-to-date on the latest advancements in plastic surgery techniques.

All surgeons who are members of the American Society of Plastic Surgeons (ASPS) have undergone their training at accredited institutions. In addition, the ASPS requires documentation that each of its members has kept up with continuing medical education courses, including in the areas of ethics and patient safety.

Licensure

In order to practice medicine, all doctors must be licensed by the state in which their practice is located. A license to practice medicine is usually granted only to medical school graduates who have passed a comprehensive exam. A state license allows the physician to practice medicine only within that particular state. If a doctor moves to a new state or opens a satellite office in a neighboring state, he or she must acquire a new license for that state.

How can you find out if a plastic surgeon is licensed in your state? You can verify licensure with your state's medical board, where you also can investigate any complaints made or disciplinary actions taken against your surgeon. You can find a complete list of state medical boards with links to their individual Web sites on the Federation of State Medical Boards Web site (www.fsmb.org/directory_smb.html).

Board Certification: Why It's Important

You've probably heard that it's important to choose a plastic surgeon who is "board certified." But why is it so important, and what does that mean? Board certification indicates that in addition to fulfilling the educational and training requirements necessary to become a licensed physician, a doctor has made a voluntary commitment to lifelong learning within a specialized field of medicine, such as plastic surgery.

Board certification is offered in twenty-four specialties through the member boards of the American Board of Medical Specialties (ABMS). For instance, a doctor can earn board certification within the field of dermatology, obstetrics and gynecology, surgery, or plastic surgery, among others. Therefore, just because a doctor is board certified doesn't mean that he or she has expertise in plastic surgery. That's why it's critical to make sure that your doctor is board certified specifically in the field of plastic surgery. The American Board of Plastic Surgery (ABPS) is the only board authorized to offer certification in plastic surgery.

To become board certified, a plastic surgeon must have completed a residency program in both general surgery and plastic surgery and passed comprehensive written and oral exams. Board certification is granted only after a physician has passed the exams. To maintain certification, plastic surgeons must participate in a program of continuous professional development and must continually meet the moral and ethical standards set by the ABPS.

Board certification is a completely voluntary process. It is not required in order to perform plastic surgery. However, choosing a plastic surgeon who meets the stringent standards set by an independent board may give you additional peace of mind. You can verify that a plastic surgeon is board certified on the ABMS Web site (www.abms.org).

There are a few caveats about board certification. Be aware that some doctors claim to be "certified" by organizations other than the ABPS. However, these organizations don't have the same rigorous requirements and therefore don't provide you with the same assurance that a physician has expertise in plastic surgery. Also, it's important to understand that many states permit any licensed physician to perform "cosmetic surgery" even if he or she is not a trained plastic surgeon. To ensure your safety, it's best to limit your search to board-certified plastic surgeons.

Experience in Plastic Surgery after Weight Loss

In addition to board certification, you should seek out surgeons who have experience performing post–weight loss plastic surgery procedures. When you've experienced massive weight loss, you may have special issues or concerns that need to be addressed. Surgeons who routinely operate on weight loss patients have a better understanding of these needs and will achieve a better outcome. Fortunately, a growing number of physicians are adding post–weight loss procedures to their repertoire, and some are choosing to specialize in this type of surgery.

How much experience is necessary? You may have heard that you can gauge a surgeon's expertise by asking how often he or she performs the procedures that interest you. Unfortunately, there is no magic number that indicates adequate expertise. As a rule of thumb, look for a surgeon who regularly performs the procedures you are considering on a monthly basis.

A number of organizations exist that can help direct you to a plastic surgeon who is experienced in bariatric plastic surgery. ObesityHelp.com (www.obesityhelp.com) is a large online community of weight loss patients that keeps an extensive database of plastic surgeons dedicated to bariatric plastic surgery. The American Society of Bariatric Plastic Surgeons (www.asbps.org), which was established by plastic surgeons who specialize in body contouring surgery specifically for the needs of weight loss patients, also has a physician finder feature.

The Surgical Team

When your operation takes place, your surgeon will be accompanied by a surgical team that may include nurses, surgical assistants, and a person who administers anesthesia. To ensure your safety, you may want to inquire about the credentials of the person handling the anesthesia portion of your procedure. Anesthesia should only be administered by a board-certified physician anesthesiologist or by a certified registered nurse anesthetist. These professionals have completed specialized training that qualifies them to administer anesthesia and to monitor your well-being during your surgery.

The Surgical Center

Plastic surgery after weight loss can be performed in a variety of settings, including hospitals, outpatient surgery centers, and office-based surgical suites. Since most post–weight loss procedures are considered major surgery, they usually take place in hospitals or outpatient surgery centers. These surgical settings typically offer more extensive recovery facilities than office-based suites.

No matter which surgical setting is used for your procedure, be sure to check that the facility is accredited, which means that it meets rigorous national standards for quality and safety. To become accredited, a surgery facility must meet requirements regarding surgeon credentials, personnel experience, equipment, and overall safety in the operating room.

Accreditation is offered by a number of organizations, including the American Association for the Accreditation of Ambulatory Surgery Facilities, the Accreditation Association for Ambulatory Health Care, the Joint Commission on Accreditation of Health Care Organizations, and Medicare. Depending on the state in which the facility is located, accreditation may be voluntary or mandatory. However, choosing an accredited facility that meets stringent safety requirements may add to your peace of mind.

Traveling Out of Town for Surgery

In some instances, you may want to consider choosing a plastic surgeon who isn't located in your area. Keep in mind that traveling out of town for surgery will require additional preparation. For instance, you'll need to find hotel accommodations for your initial recovery period so that you may be monitored closely. In many cases, surgeons who routinely work with out-of-town patients may have administrative staff who are trained to coordinate such plans and arrange appropriate accommodations for your recovery.

Remember that choosing a plastic surgeon who isn't local can present certain challenges. That's because the surgery process is just that—a process—rather than a one-day event. You'll have to meet with your surgeon once or twice prior to surgery and then several times after your procedure for routine follow-up. To ensure the best outcome, it's critical that you go to these appointments. But if your surgeon is in a distant town or even in another state, it may be too inconvenient.

Having surgery out of town also presents some safety concerns. In the rare event that you develop complications once you return home, you may not be able to return quickly enough to your surgeon for treatment. To prevent this kind of scenario, it may be a good idea to coordinate your follow-up care with a local physician before you have surgery. Once again, surgeons who regularly treat patients who come from long distances may have someone on staff who can help you arrange follow-up care with a local doctor.

Overseas Surgery

You may be tempted to consider traveling outside the country for bariatric plastic surgery. You should be aware that selecting an international surgeon may be more difficult because regulatory and certifying agencies differ from country to country. This can make it difficult for you to understand whether or not a foreign doctor's credentials indicate adequate training and experience.

Remember that recovering from plastic surgery can take many weeks or even months. During this time, your plastic surgeon must be available to manage any potential complications. If your surgeon is overseas, you may not be able to get the care you need. And you should understand that most physicians in the United States are reluctant to assume the care of patients on whom they did not perform the original surgery.

Going overseas also has financial implications. For instance, if you have complications or need further care, your insurance may not cover your follow-up care. If you opt for breast implants, note that the valuable warranties that replace them free of charge and cover some of the surgical fees if they rupture or leak are not valid if you had surgery outside of the United States. You also have little, if any, legal protection when you opt for surgery out of the country.

The Little Things Count, Too

In addition to education, training, and experience; an accredited facility; and a top-notch surgical team, you should keep several things in mind when choosing a plastic surgeon. For instance, simple things such as convenience, a courteous office staff, and a good rapport with your surgeon can play very important roles. When a surgeon's office is conveniently located, you may be more likely to show up for all of your post-operative appointments, which can ensure the best outcome possible.

Similarly, if the surgeon's office staff is welcoming and makes you feel comfortable and relaxed, your overall surgical experience may be enhanced. Even more important, when you feel comfortable with your surgeon, you are more apt to communicate your goals clearly and to ask questions. By asking questions and talking about your goals, you will have a much better understanding of what to expect from plastic surgery after weight loss, which increases your chances of being satisfied with your results.

3

Your Consultation

Your initial consultation can help you decide if a plastic surgeon is right for you. This face-to-face meeting is a golden opportunity for you to ask questions, to learn more about the various procedures that might benefit you, and to discover just how much improvement you might expect from bariatric plastic surgery. In addition, your consultation gives you the chance to explore financing options and to evaluate your comfort level with the doctor and the office staff. In most cases, this initial meeting should provide you with the information you need to make the best decision about going forward with the surgery process. Note that you may be expected to pay a fee for this initial consultation. In many cases, however, this fee may be applied toward the cost of your surgery.

What to Expect from Your Consultation

An initial consultation generally lasts at least thirty minutes and may take an hour or more depending on the surgeon. When you arrive at the surgeon's office, you'll probably be asked to fill out some routine medical history forms and may be asked for your insurance information. You can expect your consultation to involve a discussion of your goals and the procedures that may benefit you as well as a physical examination. In some offices, you also may meet with an office manager or nurse for more details on the surgery process or for information on payment policies and financing options. In general, your consultation should cover the following:

- Your medical history

- Your bariatric surgery and any complications associated with it
- What bothers you about your body and/or face
- Your goals
- Procedures that may benefit you
- Combining and/or staging procedures
- Total number of operations you would need to achieve your goals
- Timetable for performing each operation
- Surgical techniques and incision sites
- Length of procedures
- Type of anesthesia to be used and who will be administering it
- Surgical facility where your procedure or procedures will take place
- If you will require a hospital stay
- Pre- and post-op instructions
- Side effects, risks, and complications of surgery
- Follow-up appointments
- Costs and payment options

Preparing for Your Consultation

Spending a little time preparing for your consultation can be very beneficial. In fact, the better prepared you are, the more productive this initial meeting will be. Start by doing some research about bariatric plastic surgery and the procedures offered. Make a list of questions to take with you, and bring a notebook so you can jot down the answers during your consultation. If you would be more comfortable having a spouse, family member, or friend with you during your consultation, make arrangements so this person can accompany you. You may want to ask this person to take notes for you during the consultation so you can concentrate on talking with the surgeon.

In preparing for your consultation, consider your attitude, as well. To get the most out of your consultation, go with an open mind, and be prepared to listen carefully to your surgeon's recommendations. For example, you may think you've come to a conclusion about the procedures you'd like to have, but your surgeon may suggest a different procedure or a different combination of procedures as the best way to achieve your goals. By keeping an open mind, you will gain the most from your consultation experience.

Your Medical History

Before meeting with the surgeon, you will be asked to complete a medical history form. Some plastic surgery offices will ask you to fill out the form once you arrive for your consultation; other offices may send you the form so you can fill it out at home and bring it with you to your appointment. Key information to put in your medical history includes:

- Past surgeries, including bariatric surgery

- Any complications experienced as a result of surgery or anesthesia

- Past and current medical conditions, including obesity-related medical conditions

- Any skin irritations or health problems related to your excess skin

- Allergies and asthma details

- A list of medications (prescription, over-the-counter, vitamins, herbs, supplements, even illegal drugs) and dosages for each

- Alcohol consumption

- Smoking habits

Your medical history is extremely important and can help ensure the safety of your procedure. Be completely honest in filling out your history, and don't omit anything. If you aren't sure if something is pertinent, include it anyway. That way, your doctor can determine what is and isn't important.

Your surgeon will probably ask you to elaborate on any past surgeries, especially any recent bariatric surgery. Be prepared to discuss any surgical complications you've had in the past or any reactions to anesthesia. If you're currently experiencing any complications from bariatric

surgery, such as vomiting, you may be better off delaying cosmetic surgical procedures until those complications are resolved. You also should be ready to show your surgeon any scars from past surgeries. Some types of scars can limit your body's ability to heal. Typically, this wouldn't prevent you from being able to have surgery, but it might change the way your surgery is performed.

Having a medical condition doesn't automatically rule you out as a candidate for surgery. However, if you have high blood pressure or a heart condition, your surgeon may take additional precautions to ensure your safety. In some cases, a medical condition may limit the type of procedures you can have or the number of procedures that can be performed during a single operation.

Inform your doctor about any skin conditions related to your excess skin. Documenting skin-related problems, such as rashes and irritations, can be helpful if you are planning to submit your surgery expenses to your insurance company.

Alerting your surgeon to any allergies or asthma can help prevent dangerous reactions to anesthesia or to any of the medications used during or after your procedure. Allergies to latex also should be noted so the surgical team can use gloves made of alternate materials.

Some medications, including certain over-the-counter remedies, vitamins, and herbal supplements, can raise the risks associated with surgery, such as excessive bleeding. That's why a thorough

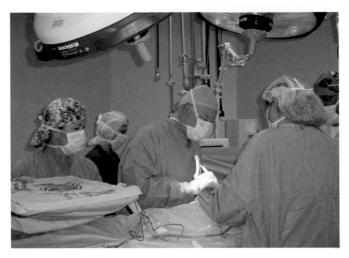

A lower body lift is a commonly performed bariatric plastic surgery. The procedure usually includes a tummy tuck, pubic lift, outer thigh lift, and buttocks lift.

Discussing Your Goals

When discussing your goals with your surgeon, be specific about the areas of your body that bother you, and be clear about what you hope to achieve. This gives your physician a chance to understand what's most important to you and to gauge whether or not your goals are realistic. During this discussion about your goals, your surgeon can help you understand just how much improvement you might be able to achieve.

Physical Examination

During your consultation, your surgeon will perform a physical examination. Depending on the areas of your body that concern you, you may be asked to disrobe and put on a gown during your exam. As part of your physical exam, your surgeon will be checking the location and amount of excess skin as well as the elasticity of your skin. In addition, he or she will assess if you need to lose fat as well as skin in order to achieve optimal results.

review of every drug you take, along with the dosage, is key for keeping you safe during and after your procedure. Similarly, your surgeon will want to gauge your alcohol intake because drinking alcohol may lead to surgical risks, including excessive bleeding.

Most surgeons won't perform post–weight loss plastic surgery if you currently smoke. This is because smoking severely limits your body's ability to heal incisions and increases the risk for complications. As mentioned previously, you'll be asked to refrain from smoking for several weeks prior to surgery and until you're completely healed.

As your surgeon examines your body, he or she also will be checking for skin irritations or rashes as well as for hernias, which are rather common if you've lost a large amount of weight. Some surgeons may check your weight and your body mass index (BMI) as part of the exam. In addition, some simple measurements may be taken so that postoperative garments can be ordered for you.

Your surgeon may have you stand in front of a mirror as he or she discusses how your body may respond to bariatric plastic surgery. By gently lifting or pulling your skin in the areas to be treated, your surgeon will give you a clearer picture of the results you might expect. During this exam, you'll also see where the incisions will be made and where your scars will be.

Taking Photos

With your permission, the surgeon or an office staff member will take a series of photos of the areas to be treated. Typically, you will need to be completely nude for these pictures, which may include views of your front, back, and sides. Although you may be somewhat embarrassed to have these photos taken, rest assured that these "before" photos serve many purposes in the surgical process.

For instance, these images can assist your surgeon in the planning and execution of your procedure. They also may be used to document skin irritations or infections for insurance purposes. "Before" photos also will be compared to your "after" pictures—usually taken at least three months after your procedure—so you can see the improvements in your body contours.

With your consent, your before-and-after photos also may be included in your surgeon's portfolio, which is shown to prospective patients. In this case, you can rest assured that your surgeon's office will take the necessary steps to maintain your privacy. For instance, your name will not appear with your photos, your face will not be visible with images of your body, and your pubic area will be masked.

Viewing Before-and-After Photos

Ask your physician if you can see before-and-after photos of former patients. This is a routine practice, and your surgeon should have numerous photos available for you to view. As you go through the before-and-after photos, keep an eye out for the length and placement of scars. Ask to see images of patients who have had the same procedures using the same techniques that are being recommended for you. And remember, doctors like to show off their best work, but the photos should reflect a range of results, including below-average, typical, and excellent outcomes.

Determining the Best Procedures for You

Based on your goals, your physical exam, your medical history, and your surgeon's personal preference, recommendations will be made about the procedure or procedures that will benefit you most. In many cases, your surgeon will suggest that you begin with surgery that treats the areas that bother you most, such as your abdomen and breasts or your abdomen, thighs, and buttocks. If you are considering a total body makeover, a staging timeline may be discussed.

Talking to Former Patients

To get a better idea about the quality of care you can expect from your surgeon, talk to former patients who have had post–weight loss surgery. Their experiences can give you more insight into the surgical process and can help you make your ultimate decision if you are still trying to choose between two or more surgeons. Simply ask your surgeon or the office staff to put you in touch with a couple of previous patients. Most surgeons maintain a list of people who are willing to talk to prospective patients like you who are thinking about bariatric plastic surgery. Questions you may wish to ask include:

- Were you pleased with the way the surgeon and the office staff treated you?
- Are you satisfied with your results?
- Did you feel like you were well-prepared for the process?
- Did you experience anything that you didn't expect?
- If you were to do it all over, would you do anything differently?

- Did you have any complications, and if so, how were they handled?
- Would you go back to this surgeon for additional procedures?

If you belong to a weight loss support group, you also may want to ask if any fellow members have had bariatric plastic surgery. If so, they may be willing to share their experiences with you so you have a better idea of what to expect from the process.

Making the Most of Your Consultation

To make the most of your consultation, take note of the intangibles. For instance, does the office staff greet you promptly and make you feel at ease? Do they answer all of your questions adequately? Considering that you will be dealing closely with the office staff for appointment scheduling, surgery scheduling, pre-op and post-op instructions, financial matters, and more, it's a good idea to evaluate your rapport with them.

Ideally, your doctor should be on time for your consultation. However, you should be aware that plastic surgeons are extremely busy and that scheduling problems may arise. This means that delays can occur regardless of the surgeon's best efforts to stick to the schedule.

Paying for Your Procedure

Bariatric plastic surgery can be expensive, and you may be concerned about the costs and how you will pay for them. During your consultation, you should have a thorough discussion about fees and payment options. This discussion may take place with the doctor, or in most cases, with an office member who specializes in financial matters.

Costs and Fees

Several fees are involved for bariatric plastic surgery procedures, including surgeon fees, anesthesia fees, and facility fees. When your surgeon quotes a price, find out exactly what that fee includes. For instance, are all pre-op and post-op appointments included? Be sure to ask your surgeon about any additional fees if you experience complications, and inquire about his or her revision policy. If you require revision surgery to fine-tune your results or to treat a complication, you may be responsible for some or all of the charges.

Anesthesia fees cover both the person administering anesthesia and the medications given to you during your procedure. Facility fees typically include operating room and recovery room costs as well as any charges associated with an overnight stay in the hospital. Remember that these fees will be assessed for each operation you have, so if you are having multiple staged operations, your costs will increase.

Other costs associated with bariatric plastic surgery include any pre-op lab tests, post-op prescriptions, or post-op medical supplies you may need. And, of course, if your income is affected by taking time off from work, you should factor that into the total cost of having surgery.

Payments and Deposits

Most plastic surgeons expect payment in full prior to the day of your operation. In most cases, you will be required to make a deposit once you book a date for your procedure. Depending on the surgeon, the amount of the deposit may vary from as little as a few hundred dollars to one-third or even one-half of the surgery fee. The remainder of the surgical fee will be due before you have your operation. Note that facility fees and anesthesia fees also may be due in advance.

Unexpected Costs

In some cases, you may have complications that require prolonged hospitalization or additional surgery or medical therapy. If your primary surgical procedure was medically necessary, then the costs for these additional treatments will generally be covered by your health insurance. If, however, your surgery was for cosmetic reasons, most health insurance policies will not cover the costs for treatment of complications related to cosmetic surgery.

Some plastic surgeons purchase special insurance policies for their cosmetic surgery patients that are specifically designed to help cover the costs of treatment for complications resulting from plastic surgery. Ask your plastic surgeon if such coverage is provided for your bariatric plastic surgery.

Insurance

If you're like most patients, you may want to know if insurance will pay for your procedure. In general, elective cosmetic surgery procedures are not covered by insurance. However, your insurance may cover procedures that are deemed medically necessary. Such procedures may include removal of a panniculus, hernia repair, or breast reduction. Common medical conditions that may qualify for insurance coverage include:

- Chronic rashes, irritations, or infections

- Difficulty walking due to a panniculus

- Chronic inflammation of the panniculus

- Back pain due to the weight of the panniculus

- Headaches or back, neck, or shoulder pain due to enlarged breasts

- Bra-strap grooving or ulceration that causes pain due to enlarged breasts

- Hernia of the abdominal wall or the umbilicus (belly button)

If you suffer from any of these conditions, be sure to alert your primary care physician or your bariatric surgeon so it can be properly documented. By documenting the problems and any failed treatments you may have tried, such as antifungal creams, you will have a better chance of having insurance cover the procedure. Of course, coverage varies widely and depends on your insurance carrier and your specific policy. In most cases, if there is a possibility that your procedure merits coverage, your surgeon's office staff may assist you in seeking the proper authorizations and in submitting the necessary paperwork.

Tax Deductions

Some expenses related to post–weight loss surgery may be tax deductible. Typically, only procedures that are medically necessary qualify for a tax deduction. If you plan to seek a tax deduction, consult with a certified public accountant or a tax attorney before your procedure. A tax professional can help determine if your procedure qualifies for a deduction and exactly what documentation you'll need.

Financing Options

In the event that insurance doesn't cover your procedure, you can take advantage of numerous financing options to help you pay for bariatric plastic surgery. For instance, financing may be available directly through your surgeon's office, and you may be able to fill out a credit application during your consultation. If not, you may want to take out a plastic surgery loan from one of a growing number of lenders offering health-care financing.

Lenders offer a variety of interest rates, and some even offer interest-free loans for a specified period of time to qualified applicants, so shop around. You can easily find lenders with a simple Internet search for "plastic surgery loans," or you may wish to ask the surgeon's office staff for lender recommendations. In some cases, you may choose to pay for your procedure using an existing credit card rather than applying for a loan.

Financial Considerations

It's understandable that the financial considerations associated with bariatric plastic surgery may cause you some concern. Considering the expense involved with multiple procedures, you may worry about making such a major investment to improve your body contours. However, with good financial planning and by shopping around for the best rates, you can minimize your feelings of anxiety and concentrate on achieving your goals for an enhanced appearance.

4

Preparing for Bariatric Plastic Surgery

From the moment you decide to go ahead with bariatric plastic surgery, you should begin preparing for the process. With the proper preparations, you can help ensure the safety and success of your procedure. And by planning ahead, you can make the entire experience a smoother, more enjoyable one. You may be surprised to discover that the steps you take now can actually lead to a more comfortable recovery and in some cases, a quicker healing process.

When to Schedule Your Procedure

Consider the timing when you schedule your procedure. If you will be having multiple procedures in a single operation, you may need to take a few weeks or more off from work. If possible, try to schedule your procedure for the least busy time of year as far as your workload is concerned. This can help alleviate any anxiety you may be feeling about taking time off.

Many post–weight loss procedures require you to wear tight-fitting garments for several days or even weeks during the recovery period. These garments may be uncomfortable during the summer months when it's hot and humid. Because of this, you may prefer to schedule your procedure to take place when the weather is cooler.

If you're hoping to "unveil" your new figure at an event, such as a wedding or a reunion, be sure to schedule your procedure at least several months prior to the event. With most bariatric plastic surgery procedures, it can take months before you see your final results, so schedule accordingly.

Schedule Medical Lab Tests

To ensure that you are a good candidate for surgery, most plastic surgeons will require you to have a few medical tests prior to your operation. Depending on your age and your overall health, this may involve nothing more than some routine lab work. If you have certain medical conditions, however, you may need some additional testing. The good news is that since losing weight, your health has probably improved, and you are less likely to need extensive pre-operative testing. In addition, if you've successfully had bariatric surgery in the past twelve to eighteen months, you probably won't require more than routine testing.

Complete Blood Count

A complete blood count, or CBC, is a test that evaluates thirteen blood levels in your body. This test is used to detect any abnormalities or deficiencies in your blood levels that may affect your safety during your procedure or during your recovery. Plastic surgeons are especially interested in your white blood cell count, blood platelets, and hemoglobin. Correcting some issues may take many weeks or months prior to surgery, so early or baseline laboratory studies may be necessary.

White blood cells fight infection in the body. If your white blood cell count is low, it may increase your risk for infection during surgery and post-operatively. Blood platelets are essential for blood clotting. When platelets are low, it increases your chances of excessive bleeding during surgery.

Hemoglobin carries oxygen to your body's tissues and skin and is vital for healing. If your hemoglobin levels are low, it indicates a deficiency of red blood cells, which may mean that you have anemia. Anemia is a condition that can make you feel tired and weak and may even cause shortness of breath. Anemia is a common concern if you've had bariatric surgery and lost a large amount of weight. That's because bariatric surgery can diminish your body's ability to absorb certain nutrients, such as iron, that are critical to red blood cell production.

If you've had anemia following your bariatric surgery, your plastic surgeon will pay careful attention to your hemoglobin levels. If your blood work shows that you have anemia, supplemental vitamins and possibly involvement by your internist may be recommended before you have surgery.

Urinalysis

A simple urine test can detect abnormalities that may signal a metabolic disorder or a kidney disorder.

Pregnancy Test

All women of childbearing age will be given a pregnancy test prior to surgery to avoid exposing an unborn child to the harmful effects of anesthesia.

Additional Medical Tests

In some cases, additional medical tests may be recommended. For instance, if you have a medical condition or if you are over a certain age, you may be required to have specialized tests. Such tests may include:

Mammogram

A mammogram is a test that uses X-ray technology to help detect breast cancer. If you are having some kind of breast surgery and you're over the age of 35, you may be asked to have a mammogram.

Comprehensive Metabolic Panel

This blood test is a group of fourteen tests that allows your physician to evaluate your kidneys and liver as well as your levels of electrolytes, blood protein, and blood sugar. Low levels of electrolytes, albumin, or total blood protein can increase the risks associated with anesthesia and surgery. Low levels of albumin also may cause healing problems. This test usually requires you to fast for ten to twelve hours prior to blood collection.

Electrocardiogram (EKG or ECG)

A test that looks at the electrical activity of the heart, an EKG or ECG can detect irregular heart rhythms. For this noninvasive test, small electrodes will be placed on your chest, arms, and legs. The electrodes are connected to a machine that reads the electrical activity and prints out a graph for your physician. Depending on your plastic surgeon, an EKG or ECG may be recommended if you are over a certain age.

Chest X-Ray

A chest X-ray provides an image of the heart, lungs, and other organs in the chest. This test may be ordered if you have a history of sleep apnea, which can affect pulmonary function and can damage heart tissues.

Blood Coagulation Studies

To measure your blood's ability to coagulate or stop bleeding, your physician may order blood coagulation studies. Abnormalities in these studies may indicate a risk for excessive bleeding during surgery. Causes for blood coagulation problems include nutritional deficiencies, liver problems, medications, and inherited bleeding disorders, such as hemophilia.

Consider Autologous Blood Donation

Autologous blood donation means that you donate your own blood prior to your surgery just in case you need a blood transfusion. With autologous blood donation, you eliminate the risk of incompatibility or infection due to a blood transfusion. Some surgeons may recommend that you donate your blood, but many do not because it is

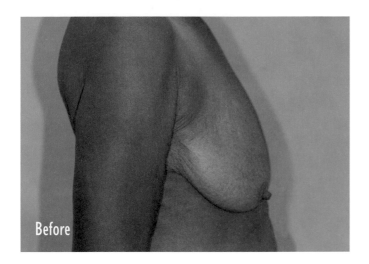

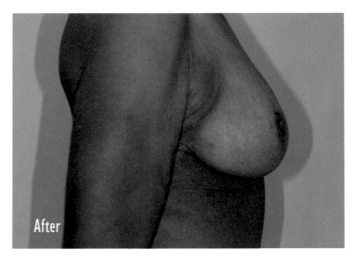

Breast lift with autologous augmentation (No implants)

very rare to need a blood transfusion for post–weight loss procedures.

You also may designate a family member or other trusted individual to donate blood that can be reserved for you. This is called designated blood donation. Your surgeon will discuss the likelihood of bleeding, which will help you make an informed choice about blood donation and transfusion.

Fill Prescriptions and Buy Over-the-Counter (OTC) Medications

Prior to your operation, your surgeon will probably give you prescriptions for medications and recommendations for OTC drugs you may need once you return home from surgery. It's a

good idea to fill these prescriptions and purchase these OTC drugs—even if you aren't sure that you'll need to take them—before you have surgery so you'll have them on hand when you return home. Medications that may be prescribed are included in the list that follows.

Antibiotics

To guard against infection, you'll be given antibiotics during your surgery and in the hospital if you stay overnight. To continue protecting you from infection, you'll be asked to take oral antibiotics for several days once you return home.

Pain Medication

To keep you pain-free once you return home, your doctor will prescribe pain medication. Many types of prescription pain pills are available. Commonly prescribed pain medications include hydrocodone (Vicodin) and oxycodone (Percocet). The type of pain medication prescribed is often a matter of personal choice. For instance, your doctor may ask if you've taken any prescription pain pills in the past that worked well for you. Similarly, if you've experienced any complications or side effects from any pain drugs, inform your doctor so those pills won't be prescribed for you.

Anti-Nausea Medication

Nausea is an unpleasant side effect that may be experienced in the first day or two after undergoing anesthesia. Anti-nausea medicine, also called *antiemetic medicine,* is commonly used in the recovery room to prevent you from feeling queasy. In some cases, your surgeon may prescribe additional anti-nausea medicine that will work for up to two days at home.

Multivitamins

If you've had bariatric surgery, you may already be taking daily multivitamins to ensure that you are getting the proper nutrients. If you aren't already taking multivitamins, it's a good idea to start doing so as soon as you book your surgery date. This can improve your general health and can help prevent vitamin and mineral deficiencies that can lead to conditions such as anemia that can diminish your body's ability to heal. Anemia is often treated with iron supplements and injections

of vitamin B-12. Extra vitamin C also may be recommended because it helps promote healing and diminishes the swelling associated with many post–weight loss procedures.

Bowel Prep

In some cases, if you're going to have a hernia repair in addition to your plastic surgery procedures, you may be asked to take a bowel prep in advance. A bowel prep is a liquid laxative that clears out your bowel in an effort to reduce the risk of infection from bacteria that can be found in the colon. Whether or not you are instructed to take a bowel prep usually depends on your surgeon's preference.

Stool Softeners

Some prescription pain medications can cause constipation, so you may be instructed to take OTC stool softeners while you are taking pain pills.

What to Avoid before Surgery

To ensure the safety of your procedure and to promote healing, you'll be instructed to avoid a number of things in the days and weeks prior to your operation. Your surgeon will provide you with a list of things to be avoided.

Quit Smoking and Avoid Other Nicotine Products

You'll be instructed to quit smoking and to avoid all other nicotine products, including gum, patches, cigars, pipes, and chewing tobacco, for at least four weeks before your operation. You'll also need to avoid significant secondhand smoke during this period. Nicotine use of any kind can prevent proper healing and raises your risk for complications.

How does smoking and nicotine use interfere with healing? Nicotine constricts the blood vessels near the surface of the skin, which diminishes skin circulation and reduces the amount of oxygen being delivered to the skin. Since oxygen is vital for healing, any decrease in oxygen can interfere with wound healing and may lead to infection or skin death, which also is called *necrosis.*

These risks increase when extensive incisions, such as those used in bariatric plastic surgery, are involved. Regardless of incision length, estimates show that smokers are three to six times more likely to experience skin death than nonsmokers. Smoking also increases your risk of experiencing lung problems associated with general anesthesia.

Medications, Vitamins, Supplements, and Herbs to Avoid

Before having any type of post–weight loss surgery, you'll be instructed to avoid taking certain medications, vitamins, supplements, and herbs for about ten days or longer. Many of these drugs increase the risks associated with surgery and anesthesia. For instance, common OTC pain relievers and anti-inflammatories containing aspirin or ibuprofen thin the blood and prevent it from clotting normally. Because of this, having surgery while using these pain relievers can lead to excessive bleeding. Other drugs that have this same effect on the blood include prescription blood thinners such as Coumadin.

Certain vitamins, supplements, and herbs can lead to problems during surgery. Vitamin E, diet pills, and a number of other supplements and herbal remedies also can thin the blood, can interfere with anesthesia, or can enhance the effects of anesthesia. These drugs potential effects on anesthesia can lead to dangerous problems during surgery.

In some cases, some antidepressant drugs may not be recommended before surgery. In particular, tricyclic antidepressants may pose a risk by interacting with prescription pain medications or with anesthetic agents. If you take antidepressants, discuss their use with your surgeon to determine if it is safe for you to continue taking them.

Your surgeon will provide you with a list of medications and OTC remedies to avoid. If you're taking any drugs that don't appear on the list, don't assume it's okay to continue taking them. Be sure to ask your doctor about every medication you take.

Stop Drinking Alcohol

You'll be advised to avoid alcohol consumption for about a week or longer before your procedure. Alcohol thins the blood and may lead to unnecessary blood loss during surgery. In addition, alcohol can have a dangerous effect when combined with anesthesia or other medications used during surgery.

Prepare for Your Recovery

Your recovery may not begin until after your procedure, but planning for it ahead of time can be very beneficial. A little preparation now can lead to a more stress-free recovery and can make you much more comfortable as your body heals.

Arrange for a Caregiver

To help you as your body recovers from post–weight loss surgery, you'll need a caregiver. Your caregiver will need to drive you home from the hospital or surgery center once you've been discharged and should stay with you for at least the first twenty-four hours. Your caregiver can assist you in getting up and down out of bed or out of a recliner and can help steady you as you walk. He or she also can prepare light meals, can help administer medications, and can call your surgeon's office in case you have any concerns or develop any complications.

If you're like many patients, you may wish to simply enlist the help of a trusted friend or family member with whom you feel comfortable to act as your caregiver. If you would feel more secure with professional care, however, you have a couple of options.

For professional help, you may want to go to an aftercare facility where the staff is trained to provide post-operative care. Most aftercare facilities will arrange transportation to take you from the hospital or surgery center to their facility. If you're interested in professional aftercare facilities, ask your surgeon or a member of the office staff for recommendations.

If you prefer to recover in the comfort of your own home, you also can hire a licensed nurse or a home aide to assist you in the days following your procedure. Your surgeon's office should be able to provide you with recommendations for home health-care organizations in your area.

Take Time Off Work

To keep your recovery as stress-free as possible, schedule adequate time off from work for your recuperation. Depending on the type of procedure you're having and the type of job you have, you may need anywhere from one to six weeks off. In general, the more extensive your procedure, the longer it will take to get back on the job. If you have a sedentary office job, you'll usually be able to get back to work sooner than if your work involves heavy lifting or strenuous activity. Your surgeon can help you determine an appropriate timetable for your return to work.

Tips for Recovering at Home

Simple things you can do now to make your recovery more pleasant include:

- Plan on taking it easy for at least two weeks.

- Clean the house and do the laundry before your procedure so you won't be tempted to do it when you should be resting.

- If your home has stairs, set up a bedroom downstairs so you don't need to climb up and down the stairs.

- Go grocery shopping, and stock up on light foods such as soup, gelatin, and crackers.

- Prepare a few meals before your procedure, and store them in the freezer so you can just pop them in the microwave.

- Have several pillows on hand to prop up your back or to put under your knees while you rest or sleep.

- Consider using a recliner while you rest or for sleeping.

- Place everything you'll need for your recovery on a table near your bed or recliner so it's within reach and so you don't have to bend down to pick up anything.

- If you care for small children or for an elderly parent, make other arrangements for their care while you recuperate.

- Prerecord some of your favorite TV shows, or stock up on books, magazines, or DVDs to make your days more enjoyable.

Travel and Accommodations

If long-distance travel is required for you to get to the surgical facility, you and your caregiver may want to consider staying in a nearby hotel the night before your procedure. This can alleviate any stress you might feel about running into traffic or arriving late for your operation. Your surgeon's office staff may make recommendations for local lodging or may be able to assist you in making reservations. Many surgeons have special programs for out-of-town patients.

The Night before and the Day of Surgery

Follow Your Hygiene Instructions

Your surgeon will likely give you specific instructions for showering and washing the areas to be treated. In many cases, you may be asked to shower the night before your procedure using an antibacterial soap, such as Dial, on all surgical areas. You'll likely be asked to shower again the morning of your procedure using the same soap on all areas to be treated.

You also may be instructed not to shave or wax any surgical areas because this may leave the area more vulnerable to infection. Any shaving, clipping, or trimming of hair can be done in a sterile environment at the surgical center.

After showering on the morning of your procedure, you should refrain from using any moisturizers, creams, lotions, oils, perfume, or makeup. You'll be allowed to brush your teeth that morning, but you must not swallow the water.

Fasting the Day of Surgery

For your safety, you must avoid eating or drinking anything after midnight the night before your scheduled operation. Having an empty stomach during surgery is especially important because the administration of anesthesia can induce vomiting. If you have food in your stomach when this occurs, it can cause the food to travel up your esophagus into your lungs. This can pose a potentially life-threatening condition called *aspiration*. Because of this risk, it is critical that you follow your doctor's instructions about fasting.

In some cases, you may be allowed to take a few sips of water to take any necessary medications the morning of your procedure. Always check with your surgeon before doing so. When you arrive at the surgery center, the surgical staff will verify that you haven't had anything to eat since midnight.

Health-Care Legal Documents

The vast majority of post–weight loss procedures go smoothly, but complications can occur, and in this case, you may wish to have certain legal documents in place. Having these documents on hand may add to your peace of mind and will ensure that a trusted family member or friend can make decisions for you in the rare event that you are unable to make your own decisions.

Advance Health-Care Directive

An advance health-care directive is a legal document that appoints an individual to make health-care decisions on your behalf and spells out your wishes regarding the type of treatment, medication, and resuscitation you want. Depending on the state you live in, this document also may be referred to as a living will, durable power of attorney for health care, declaration, or patient advocate designation.

CHAPTER 4

5

Bariatric Plastic Surgery: What to Expect

When your big day finally arrives, you may be feeling excited, nervous, and a bit anxious, too. Rest assured that it's completely normal to experience a wide range of emotions when you're going to have surgery. Your surgeon and everyone on the surgical staff understand these feelings and will do everything possible to make you feel more comfortable. Knowing what to expect when you're having bariatric plastic surgery can help alleviate any anxious feelings and can help make the whole experience as stress-free as possible.

Wear Comfortable Clothing

On the day of your procedure, dress in loose, comfortable clothing. Depending on the type of post–weight loss procedure you're having, you may need to avoid stretching, bending, or raising your arms after your surgery. For this reason, it's best to choose a shirt, sweater, sweatshirt, or robe that you can slip on without having to pull it over your head. Tops that zip or button up the front are a good choice. Similarly, baggy sweatpants with an elastic waist are easy to pull on. You also may want to wear slip-on shoes or even slippers to avoid having to bend over.

What Not to Wear for Surgery

Leave all jewelry at home. This includes watches, wedding rings, earrings, bracelets, body piercings, anklets, toe rings, and hairpins. You may think that the possibility of theft is the reason why you're asked to leave these items at home. However, the main concern is for your safety. *Electrocautery* is a procedure often used during surgery that employs a small electric current to stop bleeding. If jewelry is worn during surgery when electrocautery is performed, the jewelry can potentially conduct the current and create a harmful electric shock.

Other items that cannot be worn during surgery include wigs, contact lenses, eyeglasses, and removable dental work. If you wish, you may wear these items to the surgery center, but they will have to be removed before your procedure. The surgical staff will place these items and all your belongings in a safe place for you while you have your procedure.

Items to Take to the Surgery Center

At the surgery center, you'll be required to show identification and may be asked for insurance information, so take these documents with you. If you have advance health-care directives, remember to take these documents to the surgical facility. In case you will be staying overnight in the hospital or in a surgical facility, be sure to take a list of all medications you take, along with their dosages.

You also may want to pack a few personal items, such as a toothbrush, a hairbrush, or pajamas. Consider taking a magazine or book for entertainment, and don't forget your cell phone. Many hospitals and surgical facilities allow their use, and even if a phone is provided in your room, it may not be easily accessible from your hospital bed due to restricted movement following surgery.

At the Surgery Center

Typically, you'll be instructed to arrive at the surgical facility about one to two hours prior to your scheduled surgery time. This allows ample time for you to complete any necessary paperwork and for the surgical staff to prep you for surgery.

Registration Paperwork

Upon arrival at the surgery center, you'll head to the admissions office or patient registration area, where you'll be asked for your identification and your health insurance information. Be sure to hand over your advance health-care directives to the registration personnel so they can make copies of the documents for your file. The originals should be returned to you. In some cases, you may be asked to pay any required surgery center fees, including insurance copayments, deductibles, or out-of-pocket charges.

You'll also be given some paperwork to fill out. These documents typically include various consent forms and requests for contact information for the person who will be driving you home. Many surgery centers allow you to pre-register online or by phone, so all your paperwork and payments will be completed before you arrive for your procedure.

Pre-Op Preparation

Once you've completed the registration process, you'll be escorted to the pre-op area,

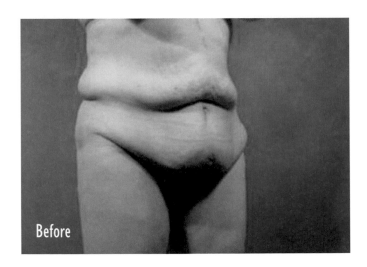

Before

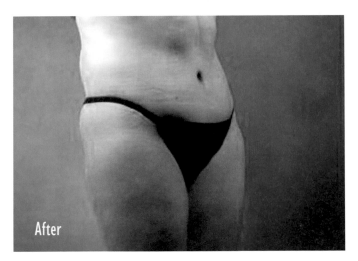

After

Lower body lift

which is equipped with beds and monitoring equipment. Beds may be in individual rooms or may simply be separated by curtains for privacy. In most cases, a friend or family member will be allowed to accompany you to the surgical prep area.

In the pre-op area, you'll be instructed to remove all your clothing and to put on a gown that will be provided. You also may be given socks with rubber on the soles to keep your feet warm and to prevent you from slipping. A bag will be provided for your clothing and other personal belongings and will be placed in a secure spot during your procedure.

With your gown on, you'll be asked to get into the bed and will be covered with warm blankets. A nurse will take your vital signs and will perform a thorough medical review. You'll be asked about your medical history, any medications you take regularly, any medications you took that morning, and any allergies to drugs, foods, latex, or iodine. The nurse also will verify that you haven't had anything to eat or drink since midnight and will verify which procedure or procedures you're having done.

At this point, the nurse may insert an IV into your arm or on the top of your hand. This IV will be used during your surgery to administer anesthetic agents, antibiotics, and other medications. You may feel a slight stinging sensation at first, but this mild pain should subside quickly. The IV will be taped in place to prevent it from moving.

Monitoring Devices

For monitoring purposes, several devices will be attached to your body. Adhesive electrodes will be placed on your chest to monitor your heart activity. A *pulse oximeter* is a small clip-on device that will be attached to a finger or to an earlobe to measure your oxygen saturation levels and your pulse.

Other monitoring devices include a blood pressure cuff, which will be placed on your upper arm to measure your blood pressure. To monitor your temperature, a small piece of tape that displays your body temperature may be affixed to your forehead. A nerve stimulator, a device that indicates the amount of muscle relaxation caused by anesthesia, also may be applied.

Surgical Markings

At some point during the pre-op process, your surgeon will arrive for a brief meeting to go over your procedure, to answer any last-minute questions, and to place surgical markings on your body. Placed with a special surgical pen, these markings act as a road map for the surgeon, indicating where the incisions will be made for your procedure. In most cases, you'll need to remove your gown so the surgical markings can be placed. Depending on the type of procedure you're having, you may be asked to stand up, sit down, or lie down while these markings are being made.

Anesthesia

To keep you pain-free during your procedure, anesthesia will be administered. For your safety, anesthesia should be administered by a physician anesthesiologist or a certified registered nurse anesthetist (CRNA). There are three main categories of anesthesia: general, regional, and local. The type of anesthesia your surgeon chooses depends mainly on the type of procedure you're having.

General Anesthesia

Most bariatric plastic surgery procedures are performed using general anesthesia, which renders you unconscious, keeps you pain-free, and blocks your memory of the procedure. A number of general anesthetic drugs are available. Some are medications that are delivered through an IV; others are gases or vapors that are inhaled through a mask. With general anesthesia, a breathing tube may be inserted into your mouth and into your windpipe to regulate your breathing.

Throughout your procedure, your anesthesiologist or CRNA will use sophisticated equipment to monitor your bodily functions. The level of anesthetic drugs being given will be adjusted with great precision based on your body's reactions. When your surgery is completed, other drugs will be administered to reverse the effects of anesthesia and to help you regain awareness. General anesthetic drugs remain in your body for up to

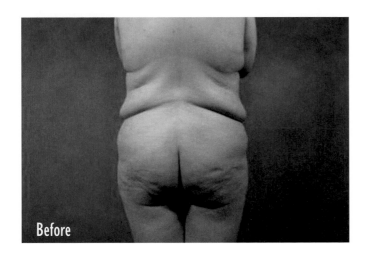

Before

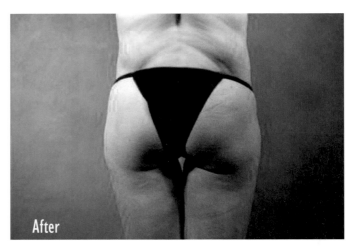

After

Lower body lift

twenty-four hours, so you won't feel back to normal until they have been completely eliminated from your system.

Regional Anesthesia

In a few cases, regional anesthesia may be used for post–weight loss procedures. With regional anesthesia, only a portion of your body is numbed. To achieve this, the anesthesiologist or CRNA injects anesthetic drugs near the nerves that supply sensation to the area of the body to be treated. This means the area being treated will be pain-free. With regional anesthesia, your level of consciousness is not affected, and you may remain awake during your procedure. In some instances, you may be given a sedative to make you feel more relaxed.

Although there are several kinds of regional anesthesia, the two kinds most commonly used are spinal and epidural. With these two types of anesthesia, only the lower half of the body is numbed. With a spinal or an epidural, anesthetic agents are injected with great precision into your back near the nerves by the spinal cord. Typically, the injection is performed in the operating room.

Local Anesthesia

Local anesthesia numbs a small portion of the body to prevent you from feeling pain in that specific area. The anesthetic drugs, which do not put you to sleep, are injected directly into the tissue of the area to be treated. For post–weight loss procedures, local anesthesia may be used in conjunction with other types of anesthesia to control pain during and after surgery.

Monitored Anesthesia Care (MAC)

With MAC, pain relievers and sedatives are delivered intravenously to minimize pain and to induce relaxation and drowsiness. Although MAC causes drowsiness, it does not render you unconscious the way general anesthesia does. Because of this, you are able to breathe on your own during surgery and will not need a breathing tube. Since sedation anesthesia agents don't remain in the body long, you'll regain awareness much sooner than with general anesthesia and will usually feel alert within a few hours after surgery. When used, MAC is often combined with regional or local anesthesia. It also may be referred to as *sedation, conscious sedation,* or *twilight sedation.*

In the Operating Room

Length of Surgery

Post–weight loss plastic surgery procedures can range from two to more than eight hours in length. The length of your operation depends on numerous factors, including the type of procedure you're having, the number of areas being treated, the amount of excess skin involved, and the techniques being used.

Positioning Your Body for Surgery

Depending on the procedure you're having, your body may be positioned in a variety of ways on the operating table. For example, you may be placed on your back, on your side, or on your stomach. If you are having multiple areas treated, your body may need to be repositioned during surgery. Rest assured that this will be done with great care in order to protect the areas that have already been treated. If repositioning is necessary, your surgeon will take this into consideration when devising a logical sequence for performing your procedure.

Disinfecting the Surgical Site

Before your surgeon makes any incisions on your body, your skin will be cleansed and disinfected with an antiseptic, such as Betadine, a solution containing iodine. If you are allergic to iodine, another cleansing agent can be used. Once your skin is thoroughly cleansed, your body will be covered with sterile surgical drapes so that only the area to be treated will be left visible. These sterile drapes help prevent bacteria from reaching the surgical site and also help keep your body warm.

Preventing Heat Loss

Preventing heat loss is one of the main concerns in the operating room, which tends to be kept cool. To maintain your core body temperature, only the area being treated will be exposed. If you are having multiple procedures, such as a breast lift and a tummy tuck, your surgeon may keep your breasts and upper body draped while doing the tummy tuck and then will cover your abdomen while performing the breast lift. Other measures, such as warming pads or blankets, also may be used to keep your body temperature from dropping. Some hospitals will make sure you are kept in a warm room with a blanket or warming gown prior to surgery.

Preventing Blood Clots

Because one of the risks of surgery is the formation of blood clots in the legs, precautionary measures are taken to prevent this from happening. Typically, soft compression sleeves will be wrapped snugly around your lower legs during your procedure. Known as sequential compression devices (SCDs), these "stockings" inflate and deflate gently to improve circulation and to prevent blood from pooling in the legs. Also, you may be asked to do certain leg exercises or massages once you are home to help minimize the risk of blood clots after surgery. Blood clots, which also are referred to as *deep venous thrombosis (DVT)*, can travel through the veins and lodge in the lungs, creating a very rare but life-threatening condition called *pulmonary embolism.*

Urinary Catheters

For procedures that last more than about four hours, a urinary catheter may be inserted. Known as a Foley catheter, this narrow, sterile tube is led up the urethra into the bladder to drain urine. The catheter may be removed following your procedure or may remain in place overnight if you're staying in the hospital.

Undergoing Your Procedure

To begin your procedure, local anesthetics will likely be injected into the area to be treated. These agents typically contain *epinephrine,* a drug that causes the blood vessels to shrink, which minimizes blood loss when incisions are made. Then, using the markings that were made on your skin as guidelines, your surgeon will make an incision in the skin.

Your surgeon will cut away the excess skin, along with fatty tissue directly beneath the skin, which is called the *subcutaneous* layer. The excised tissue can weigh anywhere from a few pounds up to about 35 pounds, but often falls between about two and ten pounds. In most cases, the excess skin is discarded as medical waste, but in some instances, it may be sent to a pathology lab for evaluation. With some breast procedures, for instance, tissue may be sent to a lab to check for breast cancer.

With some procedures, your surgeon also may tighten underlying muscles in addition to removing excess skin. The tightening of deep muscle tissue is known as *plication* and commonly involves muscles in the abdomen or in the neck. Plication is typically performed by suturing the muscles and can greatly enhance the improvements to your contours.

Liposuction

In some cases, your surgeon also may perform liposuction during your procedure to remove stubborn pockets of fat that have not responded to diet or exercise. It's important to understand that liposuction is not used as a primary technique for post–weight loss procedures. Since liposuction treats fat but not excess skin, it can actually worsen the appearance of hanging skin if it is the only treatment performed. Because of this, it's likely that liposuction will be used only as a complementary treatment to the removal of excess skin.

In some cases, liposuction may be performed as part of staged procedures. In this case, liposuction would typically be performed in the first procedure, with a lift performed in a follow-up procedure. For instance, liposuction on your thighs may be performed in an initial procedure, and then a thigh lift would be performed in a subsequent procedure. In other cases, minimal liposuction may be performed at the same time as your skin removal procedure as a way to fine-tune your results.

To perform liposuction, your surgeon will typically prepare the fat cells for removal by injecting *tumescent fluid,* a solution containing Lidocaine, epinephrine, and other fluids. In some cases, an ultrasonic probe may be used to liquefy the fat cells, which facilitates their removal. After this, the surgeon inserts a narrow metal tube called a *cannula,* which is attached to a vacuum. The cannula is passed back and forth beneath the skin, and the fat cells are suctioned out. Your surgeon continues suctioning fat until the desired contours are achieved.

Controlling Blood Loss

Surgeons perform post–weight loss procedures with the utmost care and precision in an effort to minimize blood loss. Choosing to stage procedures rather than having a lengthy all-in-one body lift also can help minimize blood loss. With staged procedures, you spend less time in the operating room, and you have fewer areas being treated and thus exposed to blood loss. In addition, as mentioned previously, the use of epinephrine helps diminish the loss of blood.

When necessary, however, several sophisticated techniques can be used to stop bleeding during surgery:

- Electrocautery uses an electric current to cause small blood vessels to coagulate.

- Suturing is typically reserved for stopping the bleeding associated with larger blood vessels.

- Tissue glue may be used to seal incisions and stop minor bleeding.

In the vast majority of cases, the amount of blood loss during post–weight loss surgery is not a cause for concern. In fact, it is rare to experience excessive blood loss that requires a transfusion.

Insertion of Drains

Many bariatric plastic surgery procedures require the insertion of drains to prevent fluid buildup beneath the skin. Depending on the type of procedure you're having, you may need two or more drains. In general, the more extensive your procedure, the more drains you will need. Drain insertion involves placing a small, pliable tube under the skin near the incision and attaching it to a small plastic bulb that remains on the outside of your body. The bulb uses suction to draw fluids out of the treated area.

Fluid collection is a common concern with many post–weight loss procedures. That's because removing excess skin and tightening the remaining skin requires the surgeon to separate the skin from the underlying tissues. In some ways, it's very much like lifting a sheet off a bed and then pulling it tight around the mattress to make it look smooth. This procedure is called *undermining,* and it often leads to the collection of fluid in the area.

When fluid collects under the skin, it's called a *seroma.* A seroma may adversely affect the healing process and may become infected. With the use of drains, fluid is suctioned out of the undermined areas, and these problems can usually be avoided.

Insertion of a Pain Pump

To provide post-operative pain relief, your surgeon may insert a *pain pump.* Also called a *pain relief ball,* this device is composed of a small catheter that is implanted in the incision site. The catheter is attached to a small high-tech balloon that is filled with local anesthetic agents. The anesthetic drugs drip continuously from the balloon, through the catheter, and into the surgical site for continuous pain relief. A pain pump can provide localized pain relief for up to five days after your procedure and can dramatically reduce the amount of prescription pain medication needed during your recovery.

Closing the Incisions

When your procedure has been completed, your surgeon will close the incisions. Closing incisions typically involves the use of sutures and also may involve other materials. In most cases, your incisions will be closed in layers. For instance, the deep fatty tissue may be closed first, then the layer of deep skin that sits below the surface may be closed next, and finally, the visible skin itself will be closed. Closing incisions in layers provides additional support to healing tissues.

Several types of sutures may be used to close incisions, including permanent, absorbable, and nonabsorbable varieties. Permanent sutures are typically placed in deep tissues and are not visible to the eye. They remain in place to provide support to tissues as they heal. Absorbable sutures—often used in the layer just below the skin's surface—dissolve on their own and do not require removal in your surgeon's office. Nonabsorbable sutures, which may be used in some cases on the surface of the skin, do require removal during an office visit. Often, the kind of suture chosen is a matter of your surgeon's personal preference.

Other materials that may be used on the surface of the skin to close incisions include Steri-Strips and a liquid skin adhesive, which also may be called tissue glue. Steri-Strips are small strips of adhesive tape that are placed on the surface of the skin to provide extra support. Steri-Strips usually peel off on their own in about one to two weeks. A liquid skin adhesive may be applied to the surface of the skin to strengthen closures. Some surgeons prefer tissue glue because it is an antibacterial that also repels water and may reduce the incision's exposure to germs. Tissue glue typically peels off on its own within a few weeks.

After your incisions have been closed, gauze dressings will be applied to protect the area. The dressings also are used to absorb any drainage of blood or fluids, which is common during the first few days after surgery.

Compression Garments

At the end of your procedure, you may be placed in an elastic binder that provides support to the treated area. Compression garments are used to improve circulation, reduce swelling, and accelerate the overall recovery process. Binders are commonly used for procedures such as tummy tucks.

In the Recovery Room

After your surgery, you will be taken to the recovery room, which also may be called the *post-operative anesthesia care unit* (PACU). In the PACU, you will continue to be monitored by the anesthesiologist and by a trained recovery room nurse. The anesthesiologist may give you oxygen to help you awaken from anesthesia and will remain with you until you have regained consciousness. As you emerge from anesthesia, your vital signs will continue to be monitored closely. In addition, the recovery room nurse will examine your dressings and drains periodically to make sure there are no problems.

Typically, you'll stay in the recovery room for about an hour. From there, you'll either move to a hospital room for an overnight stay or be discharged to the care of a responsible adult who may be driving you home or taking you to an aftercare facility.

Side Effects of Anesthesia

In the recovery room, you may experience minor side effects from the anesthesia. For instance, you may awaken from anesthesia feeling chilly or shivering. Since this is a common occurrence following exposure to anesthesia, the recovery room staff will cover you with warm blankets as a preventive measure. In some cases, you may feel nauseated as a result of the anesthesia. If so, inform the recovery room nurse, and you will be given anti-nausea medication.

Other possible side effects you may experience include a dry mouth or an irritated throat. Be sure to let the recovery room nurse know about either of these conditions. To alleviate a dry mouth, you may be given ice chips. Soreness in the throat may be due to the insertion of a breathing tube and should disappear in a day or two. In the meantime, it's best to drink plenty of fluids and try a throat lozenge.

Your Hospital Stay

In some cases, your surgeon may recommend a hospital stay following your procedure. Depending on the type of procedure you're having, you may need to spend one to four days in the hospital. In most cases, you'll only need to spend a night or two in the hospital, but if you're having an extensive procedure, a longer stay may be necessary. Rest assured that your doctor will write detailed orders for the nursing staff regarding your post-operative care.

Monitoring Your Health

To ensure your safety, the nursing staff will regularly monitor your blood pressure, temperature, and heart rate. They also will change your dressings and empty your drains as needed. Your surgeon will visit you in the hospital to monitor your progress and to make adjustments in your post-operative care as your needs change.

Your Hospital Diet

Most likely, your surgeon will put you on a clear liquid diet at first. Foods and beverages that may be included are broths, gelatins, fruit ices, popsicles, juices, sodas, teas, and coffee. As your healing progresses, soft foods, such as scrambled eggs and soups, may be added to your diet. In the hospital, you also may receive intravenous fluids to help keep you hydrated.

Maintaining adequate intake of protein is extremely important to ensure good healing of your incisions. Your surgeon will likely ask you to take in at least 80 extra grams of protein per day after surgery. It is advisable to select a protein supplement that is acceptable to you before your surgery.

Walking in the Hospital

Regardless of the type of post–weight loss surgery you've had, it's important that you be up and walking as soon as possible. In fact, your surgeon will probably recommend that you begin walking the same day as your surgery, or the morning after your procedure at the latest. Of course, walking so soon after surgery isn't an easy task. In most cases, you will require assistance from the hospital staff to get in and out of bed. At first, you may be restricted to walking only when accompanied by a hospital staff member, and you may have to use a walker for support.

Why is it so important to be walking so soon after surgery? Walking is one of the best ways to prevent blood clots from forming in the legs. While you're in bed, sequential compression devices will be wrapped around your lower legs as an additional precaution against blood clots.

Deep-Breathing Instructions

Following some bariatric plastic surgery procedures, you may find that you don't want to breathe deeply because of pain or pressure in the abdominal area. Even though you may find it difficult to do so, it's extremely important that you take deep breaths that fully expand your lungs. That's because breathing shallowly for an extended period of time can put you at an increased risk for pneumonia.

To encourage you to take deep breaths, you'll be given a lightweight plastic device called an *incentive spirometer*. This simple device consists of a plastic tube with a small ball inside and a mouthpiece attached. When you breathe in, the ball rises. The higher the ball rises, the better. You'll probably be instructed to take ten deep breaths using the incentive spirometer every hour that you're awake.

Side Effects of Bariatric Plastic Surgery

Common side effects are associated with every kind of surgery, including post–weight loss surgery. As a rule, side effects are considered normal, are usually temporary in nature, and don't affect your overall outcome. Keep in mind that every individual is different, and your side effects may range from mild to severe. Side effects that you may experience as a result of bariatric plastic surgery include the following.

Pain

It's common to experience soreness and discomfort in the days following surgery. Typically, this pain can be relieved with medications prescribed by your doctor.

Swelling

Swelling may actually worsen in the first few days after your procedure, usually peaking at about seventy-two hours after surgery. After this, swelling begins to subside. Within approximately six weeks, about 75 percent of swelling should subside, but it may take anywhere from six months to two years for complete resolution.

Bruising

Bruising is common at the incision sites and typically resolves faster than swelling. You may notice that bruising begins to "travel" below the incision sites due to gravity. Bruises often resolve within two to three weeks.

Temporary Numbness

You may experience some loss of sensation at the incision sites. This is a common occurrence and may take several months to resolve. Temporary numbness may be caused when nerve endings are cut or stretched during surgery. As the nerves heal, you may experience shooting sensations, itching, or burning. On occasion, numbness may be permanent.

Scarring

Itching, crusting, and minimal bleeding can occur at the incision sites in the first few days after surgery. This is not a cause for concern. All scars go through a maturation process. At first, scars will appear red, pink, or purple and may feel hard and raised. With time, scars will soften, flatten, and fade. It can take six months to two years for scars to fully mature.

Temporary Feelings of Depression

Don't be alarmed if you begin to have feelings of depression in the days following your procedure. In fact, it's common to experience a sense of letdown after surgery. Often, these feelings surface about three days after a procedure, when swelling and bruising may be at their worst. Be assured that this is a natural phase and that this blue mood will diminish as your body heals. If your feelings of depression or anxiety are severe or persist for several weeks, evaluation by a mental health professional may be recommended.

Risks of Bariatric Plastic Surgery

Certain risks are associated with having surgery, and it's important that you understand the risks involved with bariatric plastic surgery. Whereas side effects are considered normal, risks and complications are not normal and require medical attention. In general, the most minor complications occur the most often, and the most serious complications occur the least often. The surgical complications detailed here are associated with all bariatric plastic surgery procedures. Complications that are specific to a certain procedure will be detailed in later chapters.

Hematoma and Seroma

When blood pools under the skin, it's called a hematoma. Small hematomas usually resolve on their own. Larger hematomas may require drainage or aspiration in your surgeon's office. In rare cases, surgical removal may be required.

A seroma is a pool of watery fluid that accumulates under the skin, near the incision. This fluid, called serum, is the clear portion of the blood. Seromas usually form days later, after the surgery. Drains may be placed during your surgery to help prevent this from occurring. If a seroma does develop, report it to your surgeon. The body will absorb small ones, but your surgeon may need to drain a larger one with a fine needle.

Infection

Infection can occur in spite of the preventive measures taken during and after surgery. If you notice redness or pus at the incision site or if you have a fever, inform your surgeon immediately. Superficial infections can be treated with topical antibiotic ointments. Deeper infections may require oral antibiotics.

Abnormal Scars

Even when the best plastic surgery techniques have been used, scars can become thick and raised or can darken in color. These scars are known as *keloid* or *hypertrophic scars*. Keloid scars are usually thicker than hypertrophic scars and often extend beyond the boundaries of the original scar. If you have a history of developing thick scars, inform your plastic surgeon so the proper precautions can be taken. Treatment to prevent abnormal scarring includes injecting steroids into the scars or placing silicone sheeting on the scars. In severe cases, surgical revision of the scar may be necessary.

Wound Healing Problems

During the healing phase, an incision may separate or may heal at an unusually slow rate. If an incision separates, wound therapy treatment will be required, and healing will be delayed.

Delayed healing usually doesn't affect the final outcome; however, it may necessitate scar revision. Maintaining adequate intake of protein is extremely important to ensure good healing of your incisions.

Skin Loss

Skin death, also called *necrosis,* can occur when blood supply to the skin is limited. An uncontrolled infection or a severe hematoma also may cause skin loss. Skin loss is more commonly associated with larger incisions, such as those commonly used for many bariatric plastic surgery procedures. Smokers are at a much higher risk for skin loss because nicotine compromises skin circulation. Signs of necrosis include skin that appears to be purple, blue, or gray in color and should be reported to your surgeon immediately because this condition can be treated more easily in the early stages.

Excessive Bleeding

Minimal post-operative bleeding is not a cause for concern; however, any excessive post-surgical bleeding should be reported to your surgeon. Bleeding that occurs immediately after surgery usually stops on its own; however, a blood transfusion or even surgery may be needed in cases where the bleeding is excessive.

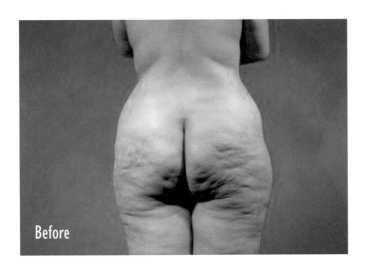

Before

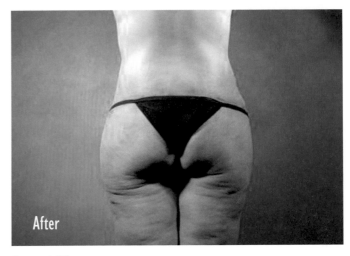

After

Buttock lift

Reactions to Surgical Materials

In some cases, the tape, sutures, or ointments used during or after surgery may cause reactions. Usually, these are simply mild skin irritations that can be treated easily. In extremely rare cases, severe allergic reactions may occur that require aggressive treatment.

Injuries to Deep Structures

On very rare occasions, nerves, muscles, or blood vessels may be damaged during surgery. If this occurs, treatment will be required.

DVT/Pulmonary Embolism

Blood clots are rare, but there is an increased risk with some post–weight loss procedures. When a blood clot forms in the leg, it can result in swelling and pain in the leg. In extremely rare cases, a blood clot may break off and travel to the lung, causing a potentially life-threatening condition called pulmonary embolism. If a blood clot is detected, it may require hospitalization and treatment with blood-thinning medication.

6

Recovering from Bariatric Plastic Surgery

Once your bariatric plastic surgery procedure is completed, the recovery process begins. To ensure proper healing, your surgeon will provide guidelines for this all-important phase of your surgical journey. By taking good care of yourself and following your surgeon's recommendations, you're assured of achieving the best results you possibly can. As your body heals over time, you'll also begin to feel more energetic. You may notice dramatic improvements in your appearance right away, but remember that it may take up to a year to see your final outcome.

Pain Management

Minimizing pain following your procedure is one of your surgeon's primary goals. The level of pain that may be experienced after bariatric plastic surgery is highly individualized and can range from mild to severe depending on the type of procedure

you have. Bariatric plastic surgery procedures that typically cause the most post-operative pain include tummy tucks and lower body lifts, which involve the tightening of the abdominal muscles.

Relieving pain plays an important role in your recovery and helps keep healing on track. In fact, trying to "tough it out" can actually slow the healing process or put you at increased risk for complications. For example, uncontrolled pain can weaken your immune system and may prevent you from walking after surgery, which is key to preventing the formation of blood clots. Similarly, if persistent pain is preventing you from taking deep breaths, your risk of contracting pneumonia increases. With proper pain relief, you can minimize these risks and speed your overall recovery.

Knowing when to take pain medications is key to remaining comfortable. Pain is typically rated on a scale of one to ten, with one indicating no pain whatsoever and ten indicating the worst pain imaginable. Ideally, you should take some form of pain relief when your pain level reaches about a three or a four. Since some pain medications may take up to forty-five minutes to take effect, this allows them adequate time to kick in before your pain becomes severe.

To ease your discomfort, a number of pain relief options are available.

Opioid Medications

Opioid medications, commonly referred to as narcotics, are routinely prescribed to alleviate moderate to severe post-surgical pain. Available only with a doctor's prescription, opioids work by blocking pain receptors in the central nervous system so that pain messages don't reach the brain. Narcotics that are often prescribed for post-operative pain include Tylenol with codeine, Vicodin, oxycodone (Percocet and Percodan), hydromorphone (Dilaudid), and meperidine (Demerol).

For bariatric plastic surgery procedures, opioid medications are generally required for about seven to ten days to control pain. In some cases, for more extensive procedures, you may need to take narcotic pain relievers for a longer period of time. Although these drugs can become habit-forming, they are considered safe when taken as directed.

When taking prescription pain medications, you may experience some side effects, including drowsiness, slowed breathing, nausea and vomiting, low blood pressure, confusion, and constipation. Everybody reacts differently to different pain medications, and side effects may be more or less pronounced depending on the particular type taken. You may find that one type of pain medication causes severe symptoms, while another drug is far more tolerable. If you experience severe or particularly bothersome symptoms, inform your surgeon, and a different type of pain medication can be prescribed.

Nonopioid Medications

Nonopioid medications are not narcotics and may not require a prescription from your doctor. These drugs include acetaminophen and nonsteroidal anti-inflammatories (NSAIDs), such as ibuprofen and naproxen. Many of these pain relievers are available over the counter.

Acetaminophen, which is the active ingredient in Tylenol, relieves mild to moderate pain. Tylenol is often recommended for pain relief as you recover because it has few potential side effects. However, if you have existing liver disease, acetaminophen can cause severe liver damage, so be sure not to exceed the maximum recommended dose.

NSAIDs also provide relief for mild to moderate pain and, in addition, fight inflammation. Common over-the-counter (OTC) NSAIDs include

Advil, Aleve, and Motrin. Although they are available without a prescription, NSAIDs can cause side effects, such as stomach pain, heartburn, constipation, and dizziness. Long-term use or exceeding the recommended dose can lead to serious side effects, including stomach ulcers. If you have had gastric bypass surgery, your stomach pouch is more prone to developing ulcers. Therefore, be sure to get approval from your bariatric surgeon as well as your plastic surgeon before taking NSAIDs for any length of time.

Always ask your plastic surgeon which OTC drugs are safe to take following surgery because some pain relievers, such as ibuprofen, may thin the blood and make you more vulnerable to excessive bleeding. Typically, you can switch from opioid medications to nonnarcotics whenever you feel ready. In many cases, this may be about seven to ten days after your procedure.

Patient-Controlled Analgesia (PCA)

If you stay in the hospital after your procedure, *patient-controlled analgesia* (PCA) may be used to control your pain. PCA is a method of pain management that allows you to administer your own pain relief. The pain medication used is typically an opioid, but it may be supplemented with nonnarcotic drugs. With PCA, medication is usually delivered through your IV. When you feel pain, you simply press a button, and a predetermined dosage is delivered.

There's no need to worry about a potential overdose when using PCA because the pump is preprogrammed to limit the amount of the drug that can be administered within a certain time period. PCA has a good safety record and is widely used in hospitals across the nation.

Pain Relief Ball

To provide continued pain relief after your procedure, your surgeon may implant small catheters into the surgical site. These catheters are connected to a device called a *pain relief ball*. Also called a *pain pump*, this simple device delivers a local anesthetic directly to the treated area for up to four days. Using a pain relief ball can reduce your need for narcotic pain relievers, thereby minimizing the side effects associated with opioids. The pain relief ball will be removed in your surgeon's office during a follow-up visit about a week after your procedure.

Post-Surgical Instructions

To speed the recovery process once you return home, your surgeon will give you detailed post-operative instructions. These guidelines are intended to minimize discomfort and to encourage proper healing. Be sure to give a copy of these instructions to your at-home caregiver since he or she will likely be handling these things. The specific instructions you receive will depend on which procedure you're having, but some general guidelines include the following.

- Protect the surgical site from impact or trauma as you recover.

- Keep your dressings clean and dry, and do not remove them until your surgeon instructs you to do so.

- Drink plenty of fluids throughout the day.

- Use ice packs for the first few days on the treated areas to reduce swelling, pain, and bruising. Remember, the skin over the surgical area may be numb, and ice packs or heating pads can damage the skin without your feeling it.

- Walk at least a few times every day. Begin by puttering around the house, and gradually work up to walking longer distances. Do "tiptoe" exercises to stretch your calf muscles, or massage the calf area to help reduce the chances of blood clots forming.

- Avoid drinking alcohol as your body heals. Mixing alcohol and pain medications can be dangerous, and alcohol can thin the blood and lead to excessive bleeding.

- Refrain from smoking, and avoid secondhand smoke until you are completely healed.

- You may need to take a sponge bath until instructed otherwise.

- If compression hose have been supplied, wear them as directed.

- If you have Steri-Strips or a liquid skin adhesive on your incisions, don't remove them, and don't rub them vigorously with a washcloth when you take a sponge bath or a shower.

- If you have gauze bandages, they may need to be changed from time to time.

Compression Garments

Following some bariatric plastic surgery procedures, you'll be sent home wearing a compression garment, such as an abdominal binder. Binders are designed to help reduce swelling and discomfort and should fit snugly but shouldn't feel too tight or cause pain. If the garment feels too tight, contact your doctor. In most cases, you'll be instructed to wear your binder day and night for at least two weeks. After the first few days at home, you may remove the binder for laundering or when you bathe.

Drains

One or more drains may be placed in the surgical area to help prevent fluid from accumulating beneath the skin. Empty the bulb any time it is more than half full. To empty the bulb, open the plug at the top, and simply pour out the contents.

To maintain the vacuum, squeeze the bulb, and put the plug back in. To keep drains from accidentally spilling, use safety pins to affix them to your clothing.

Drains will typically be removed once the amount of drainage diminishes or when the fluid turns a clear straw color. Removal will take place in your surgeon's office, usually about one to three weeks after your procedure. If you have to empty the drain more than three times a day or if it fills very rapidly, contact your surgeon's office.

Resuming Activities

As your body heals, it's important to take it easy at first. Even if you are feeling good, avoid activities such as doing the laundry or cleaning the house in the first few weeks after surgery. Depending on the type of procedure you're having, you'll be given instructions on when you can resume the following normal activities.

- *Driving:* For many post–weight loss procedures, you'll need to wait at least two days before getting behind the wheel. Keep in mind, however, that your driving is prohibited while you are taking prescription pain medications.

- *Returning to work:* Depending on the kind of work you do and the procedure you're having, you may need to wait one to six weeks before going back to your job.

- *Participating in aerobic activity or strenuous exercise:* Bariatric plastic surgery procedures often require that you avoid aerobic activity for four to six weeks after your procedure. Strenuous exercise may be prohibited for at least six weeks.

- *Engaging in sexual activity:* You may be asked to wait four to six weeks before resuming sexual activity.

Scar Management

Bariatric plastic surgery procedures typically involve extensive incisions and scars. However, a number of scar management techniques can be used to promote proper healing and to minimize the appearance of your scars. One method often recommended is scar massage, which has been shown to soften scars and decrease itching. If your surgeon suggests scar massage, start by putting lotion on the scar. Then apply pressure with the pads of your fingers in a circular motion, an up-and-down motion, and a side-to-side motion. Scar massage can be performed one to four times a day for a few minutes each time.

One of the most important things you can do as your scars heal is protect them from the sun. Exposure to sunlight can cause scars to darken in color and may make them take longer to fade. Because of this, make it a habit to wear sunscreen with at least SPF 15 whenever you're outdoors.

To encourage scars to flatten and fade, one or more topical treatments may be advised. Some scar remedies are available only with a prescription from your doctor, while others can be purchased

CHAPTER 6

over the counter. Be sure to check with your surgeon before using any OTC scar products.

Silicone Products

Silicone is a common ingredient in many scar management products. For instance, silicone sheeting is often used to soften scars and neutralize their color. Silicone sheeting comes in soft, pliable sheets that can be contoured to fit any part of your body. For best results, silicone sheeting needs to be applied daily for approximately twelve weeks, although some improvement may be evident after the first month of use.

Silicone gel is a topical ointment that has been shown to prevent abnormal scar formation. When applied to scars, silicone gel forms an invisible sheet while it works. Silicone gel is found in many OTC ointments, such as SpectraGel and ScarFade.

Allium Cepa

Some surgeons may recommend that you try a product that contains *allium cepa,* which is an onion extract. The effectiveness of using onion extracts to flatten and fade scars is still being debated. However, using OTC onion extract ointments, such as Mederma, poses no harm to new scars. For new scars, suggested use involves applying the ointment three times a day for approximately eight weeks.

Vitamin E

Vitamin E is a commonly recommended natural treatment for scars. Believed to minimize new scars, it is found in many scar treatment products. You also may simply pop open a vitamin E caplet and apply the oil directly to a scar. With daily application, you may notice some improvement in a month or so.

Follow-Up Appointments

After your post–weight loss procedure, you'll have a series of follow-up appointments to ensure that you are healing properly from the surgery. The number and frequency of your post-surgical visits will depend on the type of procedure you have and your surgeon's preferred practice. As a rule, more extensive procedures will require more follow-up visits.

If you stay in the hospital, you will likely see your surgeon the following day. If you're an outpatient, your first visit will typically be within one week after your surgery. You may be seen on a weekly basis at first until any drains have been removed. After that, your post-operative visits will be less frequent. If you experience complications during your recovery, you may require additional follow-up appointments. In this case, you can be sure that you will be seen as often as necessary.

7

Abdominal Procedures

Are you saddled with saggy skin that hangs from your abdomen? Are you frustrated that in spite of losing all that weight, your clothing still doesn't fit right, and you still can't see the natural contours of your waist? You're not alone. The tummy tends to be the most troublesome spot when you've shed a significant number of pounds. Fortunately, a variety of bariatric plastic surgery techniques are available to enhance the contours of your waist and abdomen. In some cases, an abdominal procedure may be all you need to achieve a satisfactory appearance.

Tummy Tuck (Abdominoplasty)

A tummy tuck, also called an *abdominoplasty,* is the most common surgical procedure performed to restore the shape and appearance of your abdomen. This popular procedure helps you achieve a flatter midsection by addressing several problems associated with significant weight loss, including excess skin, lax abdominal muscles, and stubborn pockets of fat. Excess skin of the pubic region also may be corrected during abdominoplasty.

In addition to removing loose skin, an abdominoplasty can tighten loose abdominal muscles, which helps to reshape the abdomen. The two vertical muscles within the abdomen are wrapped in a tough, fibrous tissue called *fascia* that can stretch and become loose due to significant weight fluctuations. When this occurs, it creates a condition called *diastasis*, in which the two vertical muscles separate.

Diastasis causes an unsightly bulging of the belly. No amount of sit-ups or dieting can improve this problem—only a tummy tuck can repair the separation. When this condition is repaired, your abdominal muscles will act as an internal girdle, cinching your waist in tighter to provide a more attractive contour.

Your tummy tuck procedure also may include liposuction to remove fat deposits. In most cases, only minimal liposuction is performed during a tummy tuck to fine-tune the shape of your waist and abdomen. Liposuction is not considered a primary part of the procedure and may not be safe when done in large amounts during a tummy tuck.

Types of Tummy Tucks

Several types of tummy tucks can be used to improve the shape of your abdomen. The tummy tuck variation your surgeon chooses will depend on the amount and location of excess skin and fat on your abdomen as well as the laxity of the muscles of your abdominal wall.

Standard Tummy Tuck

The *standard tummy tuck* is the most commonly performed cosmetic abdominal procedure. All other types of tummy tucks are considered to be variations. A standard tummy tuck is typically recommended if you have excess skin above and below the belly button in addition to pockets of fat and lax abdominal muscles. With a standard tummy tuck, sagging skin and stubborn fat are excised, and loose abdominal muscles are tightened. Minor liposuction also may be performed on the upper abdomen or flanks. A

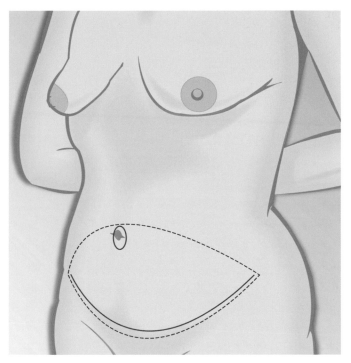

Standard tummy tuck. Skin shown within the dotted lines is removed. Red line shows scar.

new opening for the belly button, also called the *umbilicus,* must be created.

With this procedure, a horizontal incision typically goes from hip bone to hip bone. In some cases, if you have extensive amounts of skin on the sides of your waist, the incision may extend beyond the hip bones. This variation may be referred to as an *extended tummy tuck.*

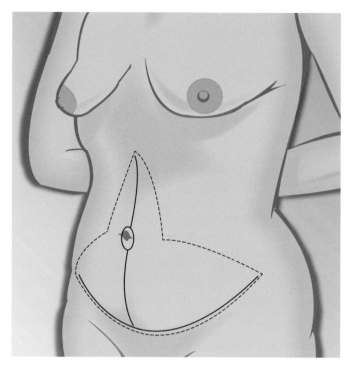

Anchor tummy tuck

a previous bariatric procedure, your surgeon may opt for this type of tummy tuck.

In the past, most bariatric procedures were "open" procedures, which involved a long vertical incision on the abdomen. However, a growing number of bariatric surgeries are being performed *laparoscopically*. This minimally invasive technique involves the use of a small camera and very tiny incisions, thus eliminating the vertical scar associated with open surgery techniques.

High-Lateral-Tension Tummy Tuck

A *high-lateral-tension tummy tuck* involves the same horizontal incision from hip bone to hip bone as a standard tummy tuck. What differs from the standard procedure is where the tension is applied when tightening the skin. With a standard tummy tuck, the tension is mainly focused on the center of the abdomen. With a high-lateral-tension variation, the surgeon places greater emphasis on pulling the skin tighter at the sides of the abdomen. This may result in greater waist definition.

Extended Abdominoplasty

With this type of tummy tuck, the horizontal incision extends beyond the hip bones and into the back area. In addition to flattening the abdomen, this tummy tuck also removes loose skin and fat around the waist.

Anchor Tummy Tuck

An *anchor tummy tuck* can remove large folds of skin above your belly button in addition to below it. This procedure requires a vertical incision as well as the horizontal incision. The resulting scars are in the shape of an anchor, which is how this tummy tuck variation earned its name. It's also referred to as a bi-directional tummy tuck. If you already have a vertical scar on your abdomen from

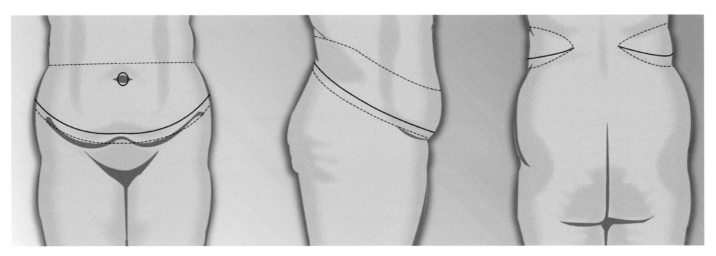

Extended abdominoplasty

Your Tummy Tuck Procedure

A standard tummy tuck operation takes about two to five hours. Variations of the standard tummy tuck may take more or less than that. To perform a tummy tuck, your surgeon will make a horizontal incision just above the pubic hairline. This incision is usually shaped like a W or a smile and extends from hip bone to hip bone but may be longer or shorter as needed.

If your belly button will need to be relocated, an incision around the belly button also will be made to release it from the surrounding tissue. The navel "stalk" itself is anchored to your abdominal wall and is not moved. It remains attached in its original position slightly above hip level.

After the incisions have been made, the surgeon can carefully lift the skin and fat away from the underlying tissues. With the skin pulled away from the body up to the rib cage, your surgeon can begin repairing the fascia that covers the abdominal muscles. Known as *fascial plication,* this procedure is performed by stitching the fascia from the breastbone to the pubic bone using permanent sutures. This tightens the abdominal muscles and acts as an internal girdle that flattens your belly and cinches your waist.

To alleviate post-operative pain, a pain pump may be inserted at this time. This involves placing a catheter just above the fascia so that local anesthetics can be delivered to the treated area after surgery.

The flap of skin is then pulled down taut like a window shade, and excess skin and fat are trimmed away. So that the optimum amount of excess skin and fat can be removed, the operating table will be maneuvered so your body has a bend at the waist. This allows your surgeon to complete the removal of excess tissue.

Once your excess skin has been excised, a new opening for your navel will be created. Your navel stalk will be brought out to meet this new opening and they will be stitched together with absorbable or nonabsorbable sutures.

At this time, your surgeon will begin closing the incisions, starting with permanent sutures in the deepest layer of tissue. Additional layers of sutures are added to finish closing the incisions. Drainage tubes also will be inserted into the surgical site to allow for post-operative fluid drainage. These tubes are secured by suturing them into place. The final step in closing your incisions may involve the placement of external tape, such as Steri-Strips, along the length of the incisions. In other cases, incisions may be sealed with tissue glue.

With your surgery completed, gauze dressings will be placed on your incisions to absorb any blood or fluids. You also will be carefully placed in a compression garment that fits snugly around your midsection to provide support.

Panniculectomy

To remove a panniculus, a large apron of skin and fat that hangs from the abdomen, your surgeon may recommend a *panniculectomy*. A panniculectomy, which may be covered by insurance, is typically performed for medical reasons rather than for aesthetic reasons. For instance, if you suffer from chronic infections in the folds of the skin or chronic inflammation of the panniculus, you may be interested in this procedure. An especially large panniculus also may cause back pain or may make it difficult for you to walk, which may compel you to seek relief with a panniculectomy.

Similar to a tummy tuck, a panniculectomy removes the excess tissue from the abdomen. However, unlike a tummy tuck, this procedure does not tighten abdominal muscles, nor does it include liposuction or repositioning of the belly button, which is performed with a tummy tuck. The results of this procedure are designed to alleviate the medical conditions associated with a large apron of tissue. A panniculectomy doesn't provide the same level of cosmetic improvement as an abdominoplasty.

A panniculus can vary greatly in size, drooping only over the pubic hairline or hanging to the knees or even beyond. Some doctors grade the size of the panniculus on a scale of one to five, with one being the smallest and five being the most severe.

- *Grade One:* Panniculus hangs over the pubic hairline.

- *Grade Two:* Panniculus covers the genitals.

- *Grade Three:* Panniculus extends to the upper thigh.

- *Grade Four:* Panniculus hangs to the mid-thigh.

- *Grade Five:* Panniculus extends to the knees or below.

Regardless of how large your panniculus is, you may elect to have a panniculectomy if you are experiencing medical problems because of it.

Your Panniculectomy Procedure

A panniculectomy takes approximately three to five hours. To begin your panniculectomy, a horizontal incision will be made above the pubic hairline. Similar to a tummy tuck incision, this incision typically curves upward from the pubic hairline to the hip bones or beyond. The apron is lifted away from the underlying tissues and pulled down taut. Then the surgeon removes the extra tissue. Sometimes, if the stalk of your belly button has been severely stretched due to a large, heavy panniculus, the stalk may require shortening or removal.

To close the horizontal incision, your surgeon will use layers of sutures. Drainage tubes will be placed in the surgical site to collect fluid buildup that commonly occurs following the procedure.

Gauze dressings will be placed on the incision to absorb any bodily fluids or blood that may ooze out post-operatively.

Tummy Tuck or Panniculectomy?

Confused about whether you would benefit most from a tummy tuck or a panniculectomy? Or do you want the full benefits of a tummy tuck but like the idea that insurance may cover a panniculectomy? Deciding between these two procedures may be difficult.

If your main concern is alleviating infections or irritations due to a panniculus, and you aren't as concerned about creating the best possible body contours, a panniculectomy may be for you. Likewise, if you want to enhance your appearance but are concerned about the price of a tummy tuck, a panniculectomy that's covered by insurance may offer some improvement.

On the other hand, if you want to achieve the best possible body contours, a tummy tuck is probably the best route. In some cases, if you have a panniculus but opt for a tummy tuck, insurance may pay for the panniculectomy portion of the procedure—the excision of the apron—but not for the liposuction, tightening of the abdominal wall, or repositioning of the belly button. Also, it may be difficult to perform further cosmetic improvements to the abdomen after a panniculectomy has been performed. Discuss these options with your surgeon to help you determine which procedure is

Grades of Panniculus

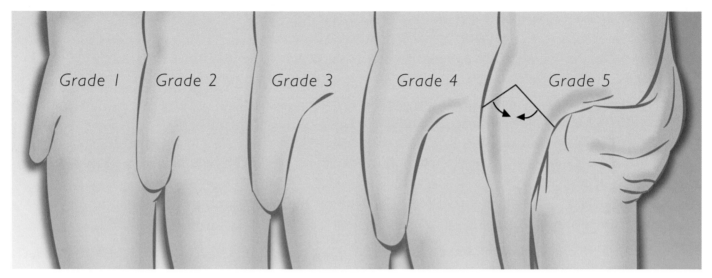

Grade One: Apron covers the pubic hairline. Grade Two: Apron covers the genitals in line with the upper-thigh crease. Grade Three: Apron covers the upper thigh. Grade Four: Apron covers the mid-thigh. Grade Five: Apron covers the knees or beyond.

best for you depending on your goals and your financial concerns.

Hernia Repair

If you have a *hernia,* it can usually be repaired at the same time your surgeon performs a tummy tuck or a panniculectomy. A hernia occurs when an internal organ or tissue bulges through a weak area of muscle. Hernias commonly occur in the abdominal region and are more likely to develop if you've had open bariatric surgery. Your surgeon may require a CT scan of your abdomen before surgery if he or she suspects a hernia is present.

When being performed during a tummy tuck or panniculectomy, hernia repair is typically done once the skin flap has been lifted away from the underlying tissues. To repair a hernia, your surgeon may use sutures alone to remedy the

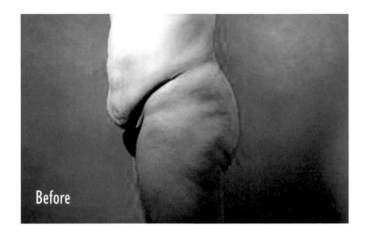
Before

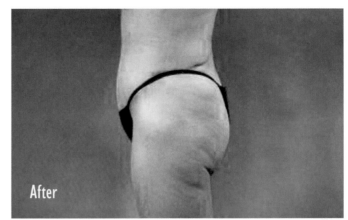
After

Extended abdominoplasty

bulging tissue. In other cases, a synthetic mesh may be used to help hold the organ or tissue in place.

In some cases, your surgeon may detect a hernia during the physical exam of your consultation, and hernia repair will be a planned part of your procedure. However, hernias can be difficult to detect, especially in people who have experienced massive weight loss. It is possible that a hernia won't be detected until the flap of skin has been lifted away from the underlying tissues of your abdomen. A hernia discovered during a tummy tuck or panniculectomy can usually be repaired on the spot without prior planning.

Hernia repair is usually covered by insurance. Because of this, the hernia repair portion of your abdominal procedure may qualify for coverage. If your hernia is detected prior to your procedure, you may want to check with your insurance company about what your policy covers.

Pubic Lift

A pubic lift, which also is known as a *monsplasty,* may be performed at the same time as a tummy tuck. A pubic lift is commonly necessary following massive weight loss because sagging, bulging skin causes a protrusion of the pubic area, called the *mons pubis.* In many cases, a tummy tuck can adequately tighten the tissues in this area to correct the problem; however, removal of excess fat also may be required to get the best result.

After Your Abdominal Procedure

In many cases, you will spend at least one night in the hospital after your tummy tuck or panniculectomy. Following your surgery, you will probably find an IV, drains, a pain relief ball, a compression garment, sequential compression devices (SCDs), and perhaps a catheter in place. You also may be equipped with a PCA device that allows you to administer premeasured doses of pain medication. The IV, catheter, and SCDs will typically be removed before you leave the hospital.

During your hospital stay, the nursing staff will provide care for you based on your surgeon's written orders. The nursing staff will ensure that your pain is adequately controlled. The pain experienced following tummy tuck surgery is typically described as moderate to severe. However, when a pain relief ball or pain pump has been placed in the surgical site, it may relieve much of the discomfort associated with having the abdominal muscles tightened.

Following surgery, your abdomen will be swollen and may feel tight. This swelling is considered normal and will take several weeks to subside. The elastic binder you'll be wearing is designed to help minimize swelling and to improve your comfort. Take note that complete resolution of the swelling may take up to a year.

At first, you won't be able to stand up straight after your procedure. For at least the first few days to two weeks following a tummy tuck, you will need to stand and walk slightly bent at the waist. The nursing staff in the hospital will assist you with early walking. You also should rely on the nursing staff to help you get in and out of your hospital bed.

Tightening of the abdominal wall during a tummy tuck can make it somewhat painful to take a deep breath. However, as explained previously, it's critically important to breathe deeply in order to avoid complications such as pneumonia. To encourage deep breathing, you will be given an incentive spirometer in the hospital and will be asked to use it several times a day.

Recovering from Your Abdominal Procedure

To ensure a safe recovery once you return home, your surgeon will give you post-operative instructions for compression garments, pain control, wound care, drain care, personal hygiene, and activity restrictions. These may include the general instructions previously mentioned as well as the following recommendations aimed specifically at tummy tuck patients.

As you recover from a tummy tuck at home, you will continue to experience some difficulty standing up straight. It may take about one to two weeks or even longer for you to feel comfortable without having to bend over at the waist. During this time, while lying in bed, you may find it more

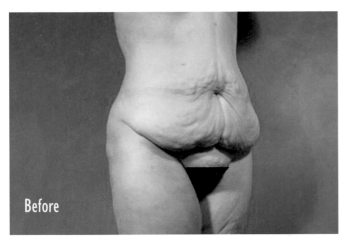

Before

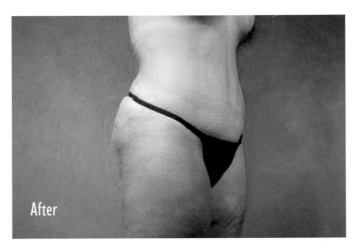

After

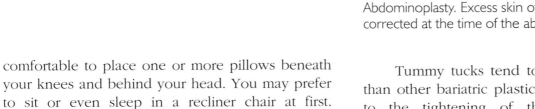
Abdominoplasty. Excess skin of the public area can also be corrected at the time of the abdominoplasty.

comfortable to place one or more pillows beneath your knees and behind your head. You may prefer to sit or even sleep in a recliner chair at first. During the first two to three weeks of your recovery, refrain from trying to pull or stretch your abdomen straight.

Even though you will need to walk slightly bent over at the waist after your procedure, walking is mandatory. Get up and walk every few hours throughout the day. However, you should avoid walking up and down stairs for the first two to three weeks. You also should refrain from bending down to pick up anything, and you should avoid lifting anything heavier than a glass of water for the first week. Don't lift anything over ten pounds for about six weeks after surgery, including children and pets.

Tummy tucks tend to cause more discomfort than other bariatric plastic surgery procedures due to the tightening of the abdominal muscles. Patients who have had prior C-section deliveries often say that the two surgeries and recoveries are similar. You are likely to experience pain for about ten to twenty days after surgery. Narcotic pain medication is commonly prescribed for about seven to ten days. Depending on your individual level of pain, you may need to take prescription pain pills for more or less than that. Let your pain be your guide. When you feel ready, you may switch to nonnarcotic over-the-counter pain relievers.

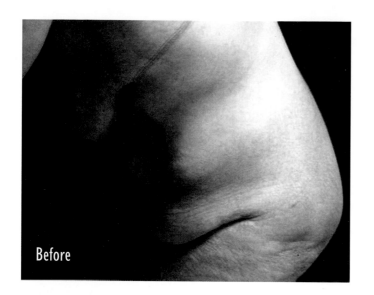

Before

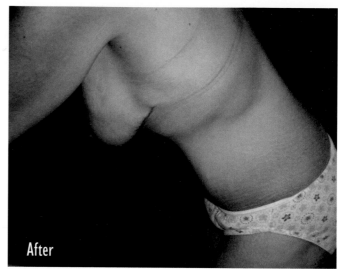

After

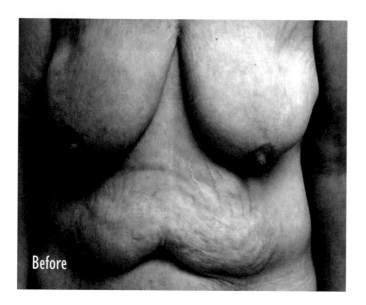

Before

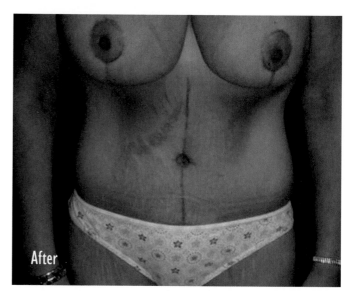

After

Anchor abdominoplasty with breast lift

Risks of Abdominal Procedures

In addition to the general risks associated with bariatric plastic surgery discussed earlier, there are side effects and complications specific to tummy tucks. These risks include the following.

- *"Dog ears":* A horizontal tummy tuck scar may form what's called a dog ear at the ends of the scar. This occurs when a small flap of tissue at the end of the scar bulges slightly. A dog ear may flatten or resolve on its own over time or may require revision, which is usually performed in your surgeon's office using local anesthesia.

- *Issues with tightening of the fascia:* In rare cases, the sutures used to tighten the abdominal muscles may be too tight and will have to be loosened surgically in a follow-up procedure. Even more uncommon, the sutures may come undone. This rare occurrence may happen if you engage in vigorous activities too soon after your procedure.

- *Surface lumps/irregularities:* The contours of your abdomen may not be completely smooth or symmetrical. Slight depressions and wrinkling are a possibility. Often, these irregularities will improve with time.

- *Belly button issues:* If your navel was repositioned, it may not be perfectly centered, and it may protrude or retract more than your natural belly button.

- *Recurring skin laxity:* Following massive weight loss, you are at greater risk for developing recurrent skin looseness or sagging. This may require surgical revision.

- *Recurrent fascial laxity:* Just as skin can loosen after an abdominoplasty, the tightened muscular fascia also can loosen a bit. This will generally not be

Abdominoplasty Facts

- Length of Surgery: 2 to 5 hours
- Type of Anesthesia: General
- Hospital Stay: 1 to 2 days
- Pain Level: Moderate to severe
- Drains: Yes, usually removed in 1 to 3 weeks
- Compression Garment: Yes, abdominal binder for at least 2 weeks
- Visible Sutures: Usually only around belly button, removed in 5 to 7 days in office
- Activity Restrictions: No strenuous activity or heavy lifting for 6 weeks
- Return to Work: 1 to 3 weeks
- Final Outcome: 6 to 12 months

problematic but may occasionally require surgical revision.

- *Feeling of fullness:* When you eat, you may find that you feel full sooner than normal.

How Long Will a Tummy Tuck Last?

A tummy tuck permanently removes excess tissue and tightens the abdominal wall. As long as you maintain your weight, you are likely to continue to enjoy the results of your procedure. As mentioned previously, however, recurring skin laxity is more common following massive weight loss. In most cases, the recurring loose skin is tolerable, but in some cases, may require surgical revision.

In addition, significant weight fluctuations or pregnancy following a tummy tuck can reverse the improvements in your body's contours. It can cause your abdominal muscles to loosen again and can cause your skin to stretch and sag again, which may require a secondary procedure. By maintaining a stable weight after your procedure and waiting until after you have finished with childbearing to have a tummy tuck, you increase your chances of achieving long-lasting improvements to your abdomen and waist.

8

Thigh and Buttocks Procedures

After massive weight loss, sagging skin that hangs from your thighs and buttocks may limit the type of attire you feel comfortable wearing and may prevent your clothes from fitting properly. In addition to an unappealing appearance, it also may cause irritation if the skin between your thighs rubs together as you walk. If you aren't happy with the appearance of your thighs and buttocks, you may want to consider bariatric plastic surgery procedures that target these areas. Procedures that help tone and tighten the thighs and buttocks are gaining rapidly in popularity and may help you achieve a more pleasing contour.

Thigh Lift

Also referred to as *thighplasty,* a thigh lift is a surgical procedure in which excess skin in the thigh area is trimmed and tightened. In most cases, the inner thighs and the outer thighs are treated separately in staged procedures. Typically, the outer thighs will be addressed first. An outer thigh lift is usually performed in combination with a buttocks lift or as part of a lower body lift, described later in this chapter. The thighs also may be contoured as part of a combined abdomen, thigh, and buttocks procedure, also described in this chapter.

An outer thigh lift involves removing skin that hangs down the sides of your legs. Depending on your individual case, liposuction also may be performed to improve the contours of your outer thighs. Liposuction may be performed at the same time as your outer thigh lift or may be staged.

The inner thighs are usually treated after outer thigh procedures and also after any abdominal procedures have been performed. This is because procedures that target the central body, such as a tummy tuck or an outer thigh lift, also may provide some improvement to the drooping skin of the inner thighs.

In some cases, liposuction of the inner thigh area also may be recommended to achieve the best results possible. Depending on the amount of liposuction required, these two procedures also may be staged, with liposuction typically being performed first and the inner thigh lift taking place in a follow-up procedure.

You should be aware that procedures that target the inner thighs are particularly challenging for a variety of reasons. The skin on the inner thighs is typically more thin and delicate than the tissue on most other areas of your body. And if you've lost a significant amount of weight, this skin is likely to be even thinner than normal. This thin tissue makes it more challenging to achieve optimal results.

Buttocks Lift

A buttocks lift is a surgical procedure that is designed to improve the contours of your posterior. In most cases, a buttocks lift is performed in combination with an outer thigh lift. The primary purpose of a buttocks lift is to remove excess skin that hangs from your backside. Once sagging skin has been trimmed and tightened, the contour of the buttocks will be smoother but also may appear flatter. For most post–weight loss patients, this is an acceptable outcome. However,

if you would prefer more volume in your buttocks, there are additional procedures that can help. For instance, your own tissue within the buttocks can be rearranged to provide greater fullness and a more pleasing shape. This procedure is called *buttocks autoaugmentation,* and it is the most popular technique used to enhance the contours of the buttocks.

Other techniques are available to augment the shape of the buttocks. For instance, liposuction may be used to remove fat from elsewhere on your body, such as your abdomen, hips, or outer thighs. This fat is then injected into your buttocks. Another option involves the placement of a silicone implant into the buttocks to provide shape.

Depending on your surgeon's personal preference and your circumstances, fat injections may be performed at the same time as a buttocks lift or may be performed in a secondary operation. Silicone implants, when used, are typically inserted in a follow-up procedure after you have healed from your buttocks lift operation. It's important to note, however, that silicone implants are not widely used and may not be offered by your plastic surgeon.

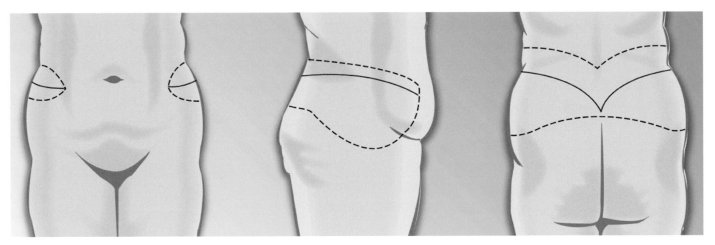

Outer thigh and buttocks lift. Skin shown within the dotted lines is removed. Red line shows scar.

Your Outer Thigh and Buttocks Lift Procedure

Procedures that target the outer thighs and buttocks take approximately two to four hours. An outer thigh and buttocks lift is performed by making a horizontal incision that runs approximately from hip bone to hip bone just above the buttock crease on your backside. If you've already had a tummy tuck, this incision typically begins where the tummy tuck incision ends and continues all around the body like a belt.

Once the incision is made, the excess skin and fat will be lifted away from the thigh and buttocks area. Minor liposuction may be performed at this time on the flanks to remove small pockets of fat. If you also are having buttocks autoaugmentation, your surgeon will preserve some of the tissue that would normally be trimmed away and will place it on each side of the buttocks. This tissue is usually separated from the top layer of skin that is being excised and consists of subcutaneous tissue and fat. This tissue will be repositioned and shaped to improve buttocks projection. Sutures will be used to secure these mounds in place.

Your surgeon may choose to perform fat injections to augment your posterior during your buttocks lift. In this case, he or she will perform liposuction, usually on your abdomen or flanks, and inject the fat into the buttocks after it has been appropriately prepared.

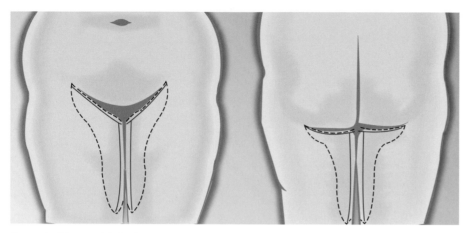

A vertical inner thigh lift is performed with a longer, vertical incision when more skin is removed from the inner thighs.

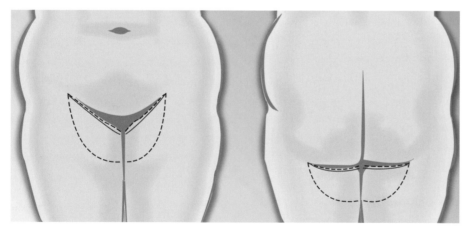

A horizontal inner thigh lift is performed when a minimal amount of skin is removed from the inner thighs.

Sometimes, after massive weight loss, the tissues that cover the tailbone may become thin. This can make it uncomfortable to sit on hard surfaces for long periods of time. In this case, your surgeon may build up the tissue over your tailbone to alleviate discomfort. These tissues will be sutured in place beneath the skin.

At this point, excess skin and tissue will be pulled down and excised. Your surgeon will then begin closing your incision with layers of sutures. Surgical drains will be inserted into the treated area to allow for post-operative fluid drainage. On the surface of the incision, Steri-Strips or tissue glue may be used. When your surgery has been completed, gauze dressings will be applied to your incisions.

Your Inner Thigh Lift Procedure

An inner thigh lift, which also is called a *medial thighplasty,* takes about two to four hours to complete. To begin your inner

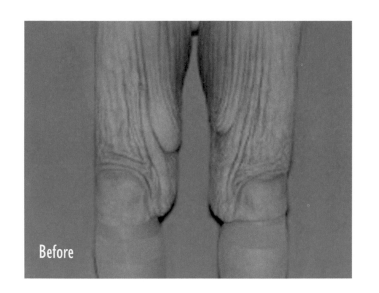

Before

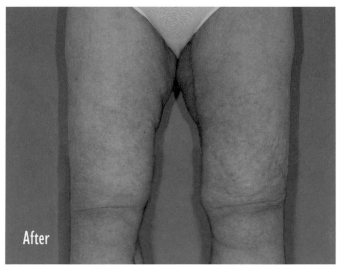

After

Inner thigh lift with longer, vertical incision

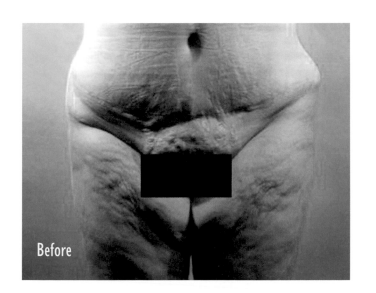

Before

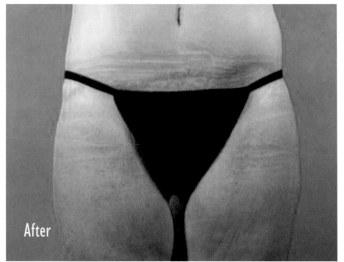

After

Inner thigh lift with shorter horizontal incision

thigh lift, the surgeon will make an incision in the crease of the crotch. This incision typically begins approximately at the top of the pubic hairline and may extend to the crease in the lower buttocks. A vertical incision also may be made down the length of the inner thigh to the knee.

The skin of the inner thigh is then lifted away from the underlying tissues and excised. Liposuction may be performed at this time if it was not performed in an earlier procedure. Once the excess skin has been removed, your surgeon will begin closing the incision using layers of sutures.

Drains may be inserted into each thigh to prevent post-surgical fluid collection. Your surgeon may use Steri-Strips or tissue glue for added support on the surface of your incisions. After the incisions have been closed, gauze dressings will be applied to the area.

After Your Procedure

Staying in the hospital for one or two days after thigh and buttocks procedures is common. Following your procedure, you may have an IV, drains, sequential compression devices (SCDs), and a urinary catheter in place. Compression garments may or may not be used for outer thigh and buttocks procedures. When they are recommended for inner thigh procedures, you may be advised to wait two to three days after your procedure to begin wearing your compression garment. You can

expect the IV, SCDs, and catheter to be removed prior to going home.

While you are in the hospital, you will receive assistance from the nursing staff. They can help you get in and out of bed and can assist you with early walking. The nursing staff also will monitor your pain and will administer medications to keep your pain under control. The pain following a thigh lift can range from moderate to severe and is typically more pronounced with inner thigh procedures.

If you've had fat injections in the buttocks, you may be advised to lie on your stomach while in bed. For optimal results, you also may be asked to avoid sitting for a few weeks while you heal. You also will need to avoid sitting if silicone implants are used for buttocks augmentation. However, if autoaugmentation is performed to enhance the shape of your posterior, there are typically no restrictions regarding sitting or lying on your back after surgery.

Recovering from Your Procedure

Once you return home, you'll continue to recover from your thigh and buttocks procedure. Whether you've had an inner or outer thigh procedure, you'll need to follow the post-operative instructions provided by your doctor. These recommendations will cover wound care, pain management, activity restrictions, personal hygiene, and compression garments. In addition to the general post-surgical instructions discussed earlier, these instructions may include the following.

If you've had an inner thigh lift, be prepared that healing from this procedure can be especially challenging due to the placement of the incisions. With an inner thigh lift, the location of the incisions in the groin area makes it impossible to avoid lying on them. Because of this, you should move gingerly and try to minimize any tension placed on the incision lines. You will be asked to change your position at least every thirty minutes—just be careful as you move.

Since the incisions for an inner thigh lift are in close proximity to the anus, there is the possibility that traces of feces could come in contact with the incisions. This increases the risk of infection. To prevent this, your surgeon will advise you to follow a specific cleansing regimen after each bowel movement. Some surgeons will use skin glue as a sealant, which allows you to shower and bathe without restrictions and may lower the chances of infection in this area.

Whether you've had an inner or outer thigh procedure, you'll be advised to avoid bending at the hips or knees or sitting for more than thirty minutes at a time for the first two weeks. If you've had an inner thigh lift and have a compression garment, you'll be advised to begin wearing it two to three days after your procedure. In general, you may remove it to launder it or to take a shower. In some cases, your surgeon may allow you to switch to wearing spandex exercise gear, such as bicycle shorts, if you find them more comfortable.

Pain following thigh and buttocks procedures may be moderate to severe. An inner thigh lift typically causes more pain than outer thigh procedures. Narcotic pain medication may be prescribed for up to two weeks, but you may switch to nonnarcotic pain relievers as soon as you feel ready.

Risks of Thigh and Buttocks Lifts

The following side effects and complications of thigh and buttocks lifts are in addition to the general risks of surgery covered previously.

- *Widening of scars*: With inner thigh lifts, scars may migrate downward. This is more common when only a horizontal incision is used, because resulting scars are exposed to more tension than scars on other areas of the body. Whenever you walk or stand, the weight of the thigh skin can pull on the scars, causing them to widen or migrate downward. In very rare cases, this added tension may widen a woman's *labia*, as well. When vertical incisions are used in addition to the incisions in the groin area, the tension is held in the vertical scars, and there is very little tension in the groin area, which greatly reduces the chance of scar migration or labial distortion.

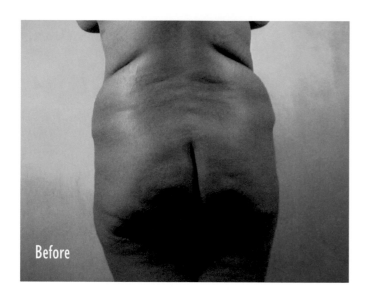

Before

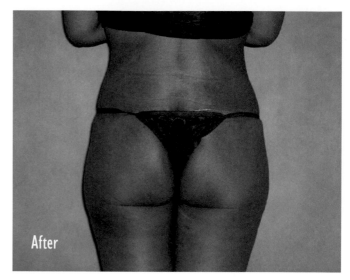

After

Lower body lift with buttock lift and buttock autoaugmentation. The patient's own fat was used to create rounded buttocks.

- *Infection:* The incisions used for an inner thigh lift are close to the anus, which makes fecal contamination a possibility. This makes you more vulnerable to infection.

- *Tightness:* With inner thigh procedures, tightness and tenderness typically take one to two months to subside.

- *Excessive swelling:* In rare cases, the *lymphatic system* may be interrupted during an inner thigh lift, causing excessive swelling. This typically resolves after several weeks, when the lymphatic system heals.

- *Asymmetry:* In spite of your surgeon's best efforts, your scars may be asymmetrical.

- *Surface irregularities:* The contours of your thighs may appear uneven, or you may notice slight depressions or wrinkles.

- *Wound separation:* With an inner thigh lift, the added tension on the incisions increases the possibility of wound separation. If this occurs, you will require additional care, and your healing may be delayed by several weeks.

- *Recurrent laxity:* Because the tissue of the inner thigh is thinner than in other areas of the body, skin looseness is more likely to return.

- *Fat necrosis (death of fat tissue):* Fat deposits may die when their blood supply is limited. This uncommon complication is more likely to occur when buttocks autoaugmentation is performed. Symptoms of this problem include firmness and surface irregularities. In rare

cases, surgical intervention may be necessary.

How Long Will a Thigh and Buttocks Lift Last?

Thigh and buttocks lifts permanently remove excess, drooping skin. However, you should be aware that loose skin is more likely to return in the area of the inner thigh due to thin skin. In most cases, if skin laxity does recur, it will not be as noticeable as in your pre-surgery appearance. If you keep your weight stable following your procedure, your enhanced appearance is more likely to last for years to come.

9

Combined Abdomen, Thigh, and Buttocks Procedures

Following significant weight loss, you may find that skin seems to hang from nearly every part of your body. Often, the main area of concern is the lower half of the body, including the abdomen, thighs, and buttocks. Procedures that target these areas can be staged to provide you with the improvement you're seeking. However, with a staged approach, it may take several months or even longer to see the sleeker contours you've worked so hard to achieve. If you would prefer to see dramatic results from a single operation, you may want to consider a combined procedure called a lower body lift, which addresses all of these trouble spots. The popularity of this combined procedure is rising rapidly. In fact, the lower body lift is currently the fastest-growing procedure compared with all other plastic surgery procedures.

Lower Body Lift

A lower body lift is a surgical procedure that aims to improve the contours of the lower half of the body. To achieve this, it combines a number of post–weight loss procedures into a single operation. In most cases, a lower body lift involves a tummy tuck along with an outer thigh lift and a buttocks lift. With this procedure, your plastic surgeon takes a three-dimensional approach to reshaping the contours of the lower half of your body.

The lower body lift can produce some of the most dramatic results possible with plastic surgery. Where you once had sagging flesh on your abdomen, thighs, buttocks, and lower back, you will find a tighter, more toned appearance. For instance, your abdomen will appear flatter, and your waist will have more defined contours. In addition, your thighs will be smoother, and

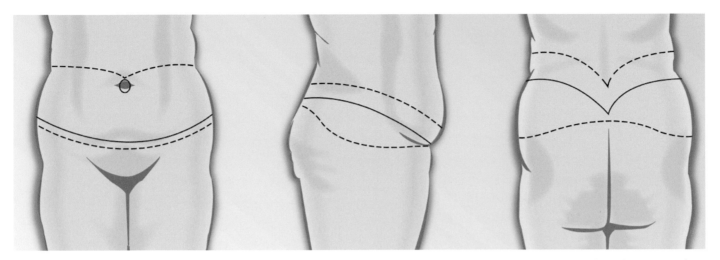

A body lift usually includes a tummy tuck, outer thigh lift, and buttocks lift. Skin shown within the dotted lines is removed. Red line shows scar.

your buttocks will no longer be as droopy. Overall, this procedure can create a more natural-looking, attractive body shape. Often, if you have lost more than eighty pounds, you will have a circumferential excess of skin, which is best corrected with a circumferential procedure, such as a lower body lift.

A lower body lift typically produces more balanced body proportions than if you have a single procedure, such as a tummy tuck. For instance, a tummy tuck can improve the contours of your abdomen and waist, but in doing so, it may make the sagging skin on your thighs and buttocks more noticeable. And after your waist has been cinched, your hips may actually appear wider

as a result. In this case, problems with your thighs also can be addressed in a follow-up procedure. But if you want a more complete makeover, a lower body lift is more likely to give you the results you want.

If you've experienced massive weight loss, the lower body lift can help restore the contours of your body. Similarly, a lower body lift can improve body contours that have been altered due to pregnancy or the aging process. In addition, this procedure can address the sagging skin that may result from liposuction of the abdomen, thighs, and buttocks.

Be aware that plastic surgeons may refer to a lower body lift using a variety of terms. For

Combined Abdomen, Thigh, and Buttocks Procedures

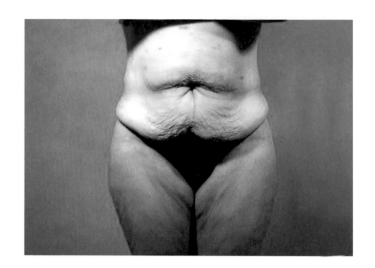
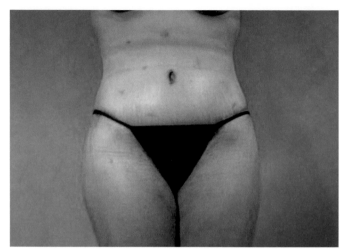
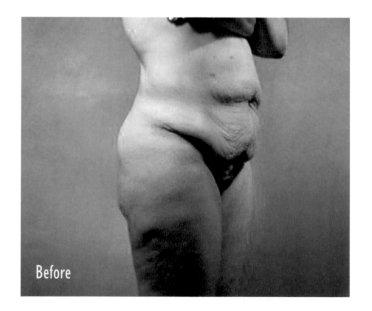
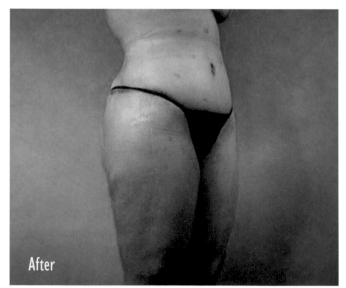

Before

After

Lower body lift with inner and outer thigh lift

instance, the procedure also may be called a *body lift, belt lipectomy, circumferential body lipectomy, central body lift,* or *circumferential torsoplasty.* In some cases, the surgical techniques used for these procedures may differ slightly among surgeons. Because of this, if your surgeon recommends a lower body lift or uses one of these other terms, be sure you understand exactly what the procedure entails.

In addition, the specific techniques used for a lower body lift will vary depending on your individual situation. For instance, the amount of excess skin you have may play an important role in determining how your lower body lift will be performed. Similarly, whether or not you have a vertical scar on your abdomen from a previous bariatric surgery may be a factor in the way your surgeon approaches your procedure. Regardless of the specific surgical techniques employed, a lower body lift may give your body better overall proportions and a more pleasing appearance.

Your Lower Body Lift Procedure

The length of time required for a lower body lift procedure typically ranges from about four to eight hours. Your surgeon will determine the best order in which to perform your procedure based on your individual needs. Your surgeon's personal preference also may be a factor in this decision.

Most of the time, a lower body lift begins with the outer thigh and buttocks lift portion of the procedure. Depending on your surgeon's preference, you may be placed on your stomach for this part of the procedure, or you may be positioned on your side. In most cases, your surgeon will make an incision that begins just above the buttocks crease and continues out over the hip toward the hip bone. In addition to shaping the thighs and buttocks, your surgeon also will remove sagging skin on your lower back at this time. Buttocks autoaugmentation or fat injections also may be performed to enhance the projection of your rear end. (See the chapter on thigh and buttocks procedures for a detailed description of these procedures.)

After the first side of your flanks and buttocks has been reshaped, your surgeon will repeat this procedure on your other side. If you were positioned on your side, your body will carefully be rotated to the other side for this segment of the operation. If you were lying facedown, your body does not need to be turned.

Once the contouring of your thighs, buttocks, and lower back has been completed, your body will be gently turned so you will be lying flat on your back on the operating table. At this time, your surgeon will begin the tummy tuck procedure. (For a detailed description of the tummy tuck procedure, see the chapter on Abdominal Procedures.)

During your lower body lift, liposuction may be used to fine-tune the contours of your body. For instance, pockets of fat may be removed from

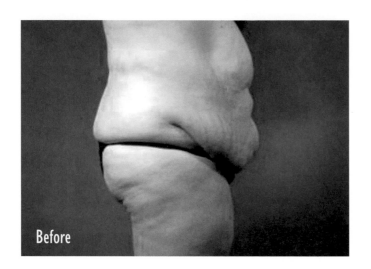
Before

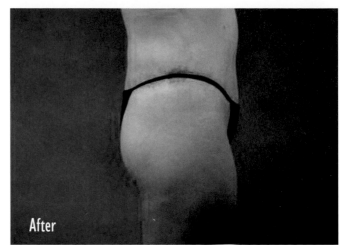
After

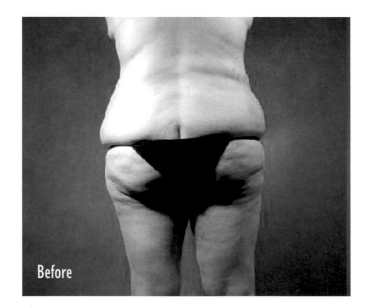
Before

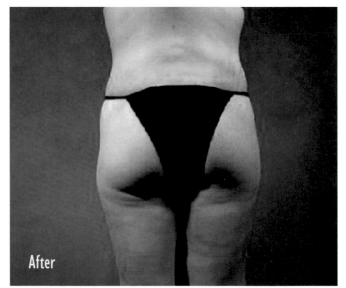
After

Lower body lift

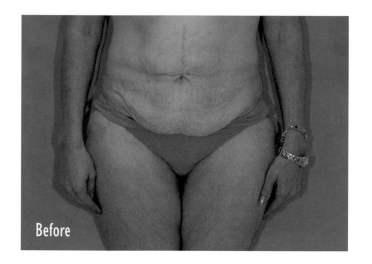

Before

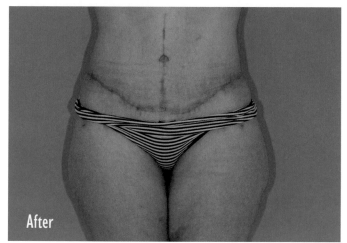

After

Lower body lift with anchor incision

your abdomen, outer thighs, or buttocks. In most cases, however, fat removal is not considered a primary objective for a lower body lift. Any liposuction being performed will usually be minor.

When the contouring portion of your procedure is finished, the horizontal incision will extend all the way around your lower torso, creating a sort of "belt." In some cases, you also may have a vertical incision on your abdomen. Once your incisions have been closed with layers of sutures and sealed with either Steri-Strips or tissue glue, they will be covered with light gauze dressings. Another small, round incision will be visible around your belly button, which is relocated during the tummy tuck portion of the procedure.

During your operation, several drains will be placed under the skin to prevent fluid from collecting in the surgical area. In addition, a pain pump may be placed in the abdomen where the muscles have been tightened. An elastic binder that fits around your abdomen may be placed on you to provide gentle pressure, to reduce swelling, and to provide stability. At this point, your procedure is complete, and you will be moved out of the operating room to the recovery area.

After Your Lower Body Lift Procedure

After your lower body lift, you will usually stay in the hospital for one to four days. In most cases, an IV will be attached to your arm or to the

Combined Abdomen, Thigh, and Buttocks Procedures

back of your hand and may be used to administer fluids, pain medication, and antibiotics. You also may be outfitted with a pain relief ball, drains, sequential compression devices (SCDs), an elastic binder, and possibly a catheter. A patient-controlled analgisia (PCA) device that delivers pre-measured doses of pain reliever when you press a button also is commonly used. The catheter, SCDs, PCA, and IV will all typically be removed before you are discharged from the hospital.

To ensure your well-being while you are in the hospital, your surgeon will provide written orders for the nursing staff regarding your care. One of the primary goals of the nursing staff will be to manage any pain you might be experiencing. The pain following a lower body lift usually ranges from moderate to severe. While in the hospital, the pain relief ball and the PCA device may be adequate to control your pain. If not, you should alert the nursing staff.

It's common after a lower body lift for your entire midsection to feel swollen and tight. Swelling may increase over the first day or two before it begins to subside. If you are wearing an elastic binder, it should help reduce the swelling.

The nursing staff also will be charged with assisting you as you move. Since your lower body lift incision goes completely around your torso, you must be very careful when you change positions, when you get in or out of the hospital bed, or when you walk. To protect your incision, the nursing staff or a physical therapist will assist you in moving, rather than allowing you to maneuver around by yourself.

Since a lower body lift generally involves tightening of the abdominal wall, you may find it difficult or even painful to breathe deeply. As discussed earlier, taking deep breaths is necessary in order to reduce the chances of developing rare complications, such as pneumonia. To make sure your breathing is sufficiently deep, you will be advised to use an incentive spirometer during your hospital stay. In most cases, you will need to use this simple device numerous times throughout the day.

While you are in the hospital, the nursing staff also will change your dressings and empty your drains in accordance with your surgeon's orders. Before you leave the hospital, these aftercare professionals most likely will show you and your caregiver how to empty and care for your drains so you will understand how to do it at home.

Recovering from Your Lower Body Lift Procedure

Recovering from the procedure takes time, considering how extensive it is and how many areas of the body are involved. Remember that your abdominal muscles are affected as well as your abdomen, outer thighs, lower back, and buttocks. You can expect your recovery to take longer than if you had only had a tummy tuck or only had an outer thigh and buttocks lift. In fact, a lower body lift is usually associated with the most uncomfortable recovery period of all bariatric plastic surgery procedures.

You can expect to experience pain for approximately ten to twenty days and will likely require narcotic pain medication to alleviate discomfort during this time. However, if your surgeon inserted a pain pump into the abdominal area, you may find that your pain is diminished. When you feel ready, you may switch to any over-the-counter pain relievers approved by your doctor.

During the healing phase, you are likely to find it difficult to sit down for the first one to two weeks or more. For the first week or so, you also

will feel some discomfort when walking. Normally, with a tummy tuck, you would be instructed to walk slightly bent over at the waist. However, you are usually not able to do this with a lower body lift.

Walking while bent forward at the waist may tug on the incision on your backside. And bending backward, which would provide some relief for your back, would cause tension on your abdomen. In general, you'll have to find a position somewhere in between that causes the least amount of discomfort. Many surgeons will recommend the "lawn chair position" with your hips and knees slightly bent. This can be accomplished in a recliner, in a lift chair, or even in your bed with the pillows arranged appropriately. For

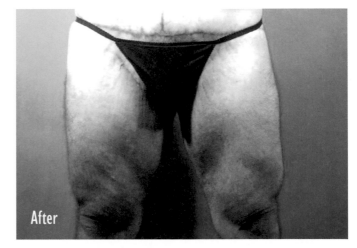

Lower body lift with inner thigh lift

Combined Abdomen, Thigh, and Buttocks Procedures

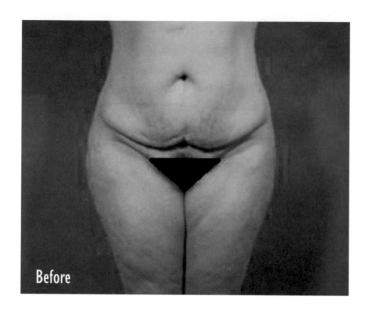

Before

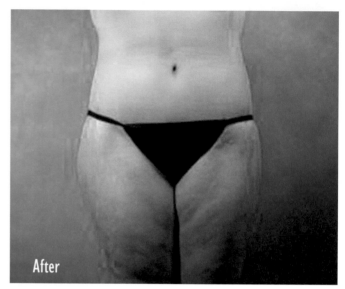

After

Lower body lift

approximately two to three weeks, you also will be advised to avoid stretching or bending down.

As for hygiene, you will be restricted to taking a sponge bath until your surgeon gives you the go-ahead to take a shower or a bath. If surgical glue is used to seal the incisions, you may be allowed to bathe immediately after surgery. Typically, you may begin showering once your drains have been removed, which may not take place for two to four weeks after your surgery. (Some surgeons may allow you to shower with your drains.) While your drains are in place, you will need to care for them as discussed previously.

Swelling following a lower body lift can be significant and typically increases during the first few days. By wearing your abdominal binder continuously for the first two to three weeks, you can help reduce swelling. If your compression garment feels too tight, remove it, and contact your surgeon. When an elastic binder is too constricting, it can reduce blood supply, which may limit your body's ability to heal. In some cases, you may choose to continue wearing your compression garment for several months after surgery if you find that it provides comfort and minimizes swelling. After a few weeks, most surgeons will allow you to switch to a slightly looser "second

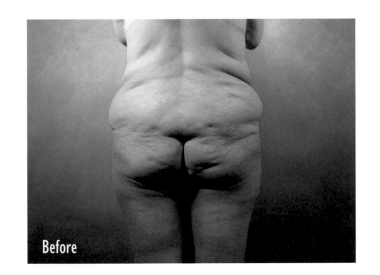

Before

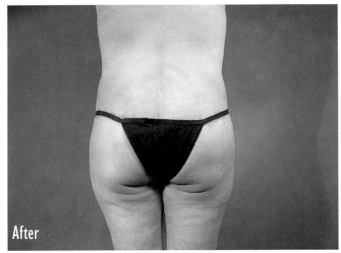

After

Lower body lift

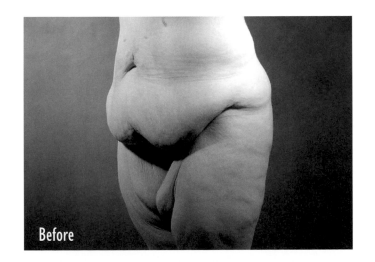

Before

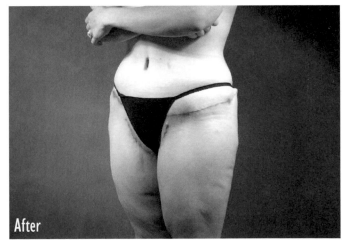

After

Lower body lift with inner thigh lift

Combined Abdomen, Thigh, and Buttocks Procedures

89

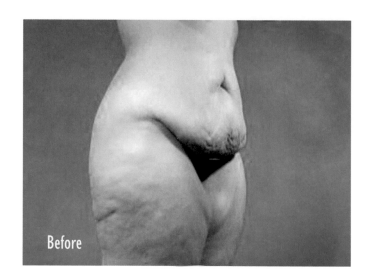

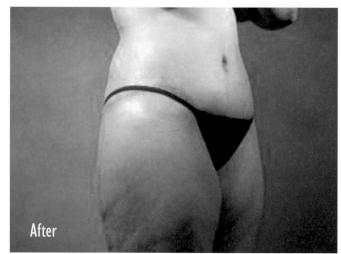

Lower body lift

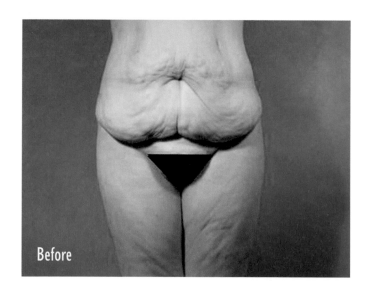

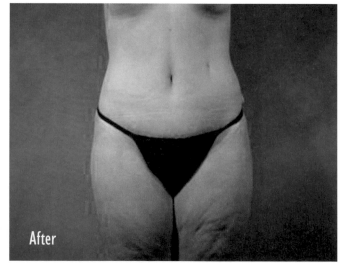

Lower body lift

stage" compression garment without zippers that is easier to wear under clothes.

Sutures around the belly button will be removed in about five to seven days. In most cases, the sutures used for your horizontal incision are permanent or absorbable. When this is the case, there are no other visible sutures that require removal.

If your job involves light office work, you should count on taking up to four weeks off before returning to work. For jobs that require heavy lifting or physical labor, you may be advised to wait at least six weeks before heading back to work. Similarly, you will need to avoid any heavy lifting or strenuous activity or exercise for approximately six weeks or more.

Staging or Combining Your Procedure?

Although a lower body lift is appealing because it can dramatically reshape your body, remember that it is a very extensive operation that requires many hours in the operating room and significant recovery time at home. Whether your surgeon recommends a lower body lift or prefers to stage these procedures depends on several factors.

For instance, your overall health or age may be a factor in the decision to stage or combine procedures. If you have a medical condition or if you are over a certain age, your surgeon may feel

it's best to limit your time in the operating room by staging procedures.

In addition, plastic surgeons have personal preferences about staging or combining procedures based on their past experience. Some surgeons simply prefer performing a lower body lift as opposed to staging procedures. For others, the opposite is true. In addition, there tend to be regional trends, with lower body lifts more likely to be offered in some areas of the country and staged procedures more commonly recommended in other areas. The type of facility used—a hospital versus a surgery center—also may influence whether your surgeon is comfortable performing a more involved procedure.

Similarly, if you have a demanding job or you care for small children, you may not be able to take enough time off to allow your body to heal properly. In this case, even though you may want the overall results offered by a lower body lift, you may need to stage procedures to fit into your busy schedule.

Risks of Lower Body Lifts

Because a lower body lift is such an extensive procedure, it is typically associated with a wider range of possible complications. In addition to the general risks of surgery that apply to any type of procedure, a lower body lift also includes all the risks associated with a tummy tuck. (See the Abdominal Procedures chapter for a list of risks.)

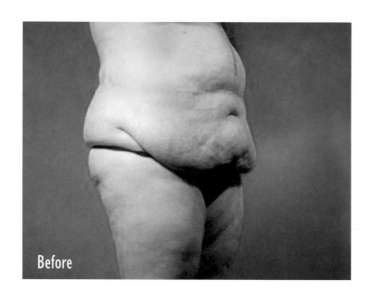
Before

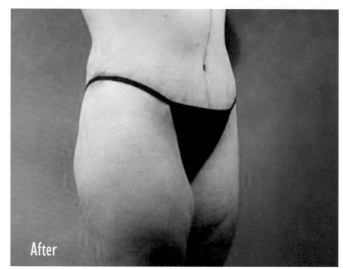
After

Lower body lift

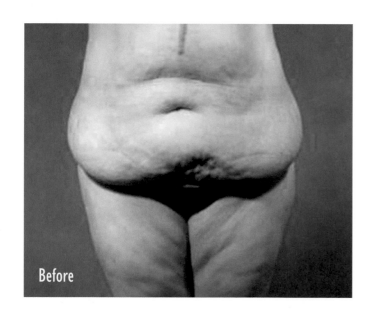
Before

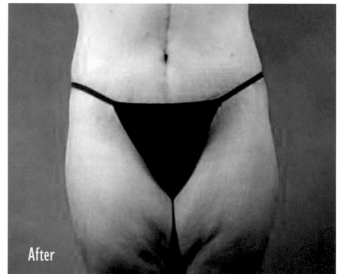
After

Lower body lift

Other complications are also of particular concern with a lower body lift, including the following.

- *Bleeding:* Because a large amount of skin is often removed, bleeding can occur during or after surgery. In some cases, a blood transfusion may be required, or you may need additional surgery to stop the bleeding. If you have anemia, you will be encouraged to correct it before surgery to lessen the likelihood of needing a transfusion.

- *Seroma:* Fluid collection under the skin is the most common complication associated with lower body lifts. Fluid build-up can usually be aspirated with a needle in your surgeon's office a few times a week for two to three weeks. In very rare cases, surgical intervention may be required.

- *Scar widening:* Scars in the central back area are exposed to higher tension due to normal body movements such as bending and stretching and are more likely to widen as a result.

- *Wound separation:* With a lower body lift, wound separation is uncommon but can occur.

- *Fat necrosis:* Excessive tension or infection may cause underlying fat to die. Although uncommon, fat necrosis will delay healing and may require surgical revision of the scar.

- *Skin necrosis:* If skin is pulled too tight or if you have an infection, it may lead to skin death. This can lead to a prolonged healing period, additional scarring, or the need for follow-up surgery to correct the problem.

- *Asymmetry/inadequate lifting:* Results that are asymmetrical and lifts that are inadequate are more common if you have a significant amount of excess skin to remove. In severe cases, surgical revision may be required.

- *Deep venous thrombosis (DVT)/pulmonary embolism:* Although DVT and pulmonary embolism are rare, there is an increased risk with a lower body lift. Using SCDs and compression stockings, along with early walking after surgery, can help reduce the risk. During the first few weeks following surgery, your risk is higher due to lower activity levels. If you are considered at risk for developing DVT, blood thinners may be prescribed as a precaution. If they do occur, blood clots may require additional hospitalization, but they usually resolve completely with proper treatment.

Follow-Up Appointments

After your lower body lift, you will continue to see your plastic surgeon throughout your recovery. Usually, your surgeon will visit you in

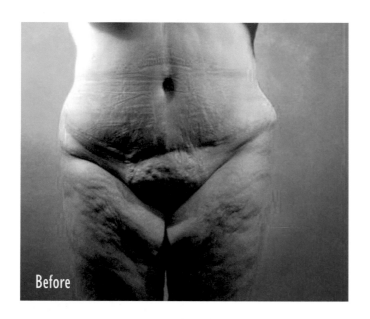
Before

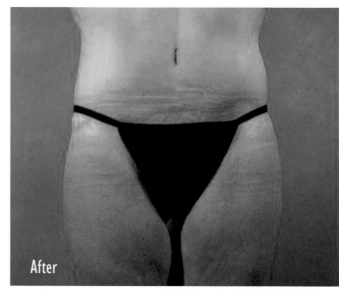
After

Lower body lift with inner thigh lift

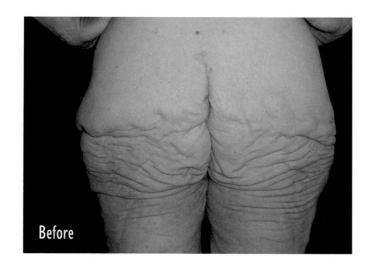
Before

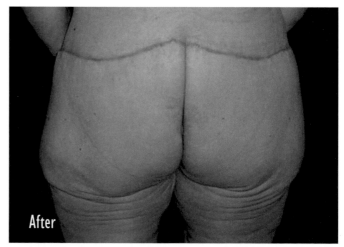
After

Lower body lift

Body Lift Facts

- Length of Surgery: 4 to 8 hours

- Type of Anesthesia: General

- Hospital Stay: 1 to 4 days

- Pain Level: Moderate to severe

- Drains: Yes, usually removed in 2 to 4 weeks

- Compression Garment: Abdominal binder for at least 2 weeks

- Visible Sutures: Usually only around belly button, removed in 5 to 7 days in office

- Activity Restrictions: No strenuous activity or heavy lifting for 6 weeks

- Return to Work: Up to 6 weeks

- Final Outcome: 6 to 12 months

How Long Will a Lower Body Lift Last?

With a lower body lift, sagging skin is permanently removed from the abdomen, hips, thighs, and buttocks. In addition, the muscles of the abdominal wall are tightened with permanent sutures. Ideally, your results will be long-lasting. However, some things can adversely affect your results. For instance, major changes in your weight as well as pregnancy, can stretch the skin and cause the abdominal muscles to separate again. In addition, the fact that you have already lost a significant amount of weight puts you at a higher risk for having recurrent looseness of the skin. To ensure that you maintain the best possible outcome, you will need to keep your weight stabilized.

the hospital the day after your procedure to check on your progress. When you are able to eat, move about effectively, and have adequate pain control, you will be discharged from the hospital. After you've been discharged, you'll likely have weekly appointments in your surgeon's office until your drains are removed. Once your drains have been removed, you will probably see your surgeon on a less-frequent basis.

10

Breast Procedures

When you lose 50 pounds, 100 pounds, or even more, you may find that your breasts change in undesirable ways. Breasts often lose their fullness, firmness, and shape after massive weight loss. And when breasts lose volume, they droop and sag. This common condition is called *ptosis* (pronounced toe-sis). Weight loss isn't the only reason that breasts may sag—pregnancy and the natural aging process also can cause breasts to drift downward. If you feel self-conscious about the way your breasts have transformed, you may want to consider plastic surgery procedures that can restore the shape of droopy breasts. A number of surgical options are available to give your breasts a more youthful and pleasing appearance.

With weight fluctuations, women aren't the only ones who suffer with unwanted changes to the chest area. If you're a man, you may have been embarrassed if you developed enlarged breasts when you were overweight. And you may feel even more frustrated if you have sagging in the chest area after shedding a significant amount of fat. Fortunately, there are procedures that can address your problems, too, to give you a more natural, masculine-looking chest.

Breast Lift

A breast lift, which also is called a *mastopexy,* is a surgical procedure that aims to minimize sagging and restore the contours of your breasts. The procedure primarily removes excess skin and tightens the remaining skin on your breasts to provide better support for the breast tissue. This lifts the breasts to a more natural position on the chest wall, restores volume to the upper portion of the breasts, and raises drooping nipples to the center of the breasts. In addition, the size of your *areola* can be reduced if you think it is too large.

Degrees of Ptosis

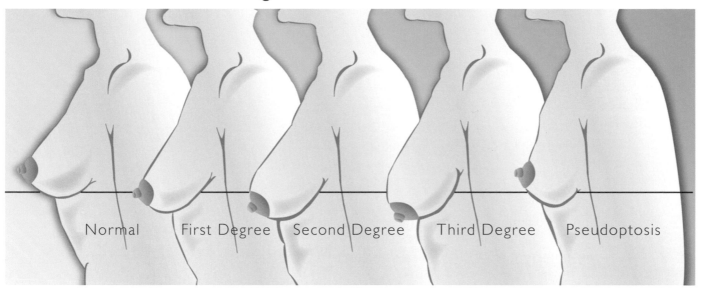

Normal   First Degree   Second Degree   Third Degree   Pseudoptosis

If you're bothered by the way your breasts sag, you may benefit from a breast lift. The amount of lift you need depends on the degree of ptosis you have. Plastic surgeons generally classify the degree of ptosis based on the position of the nipple in relation to the *inframammary fold*, the crease below the breast. In normal breasts that don't sag, the nipple lies in the center of the breast mound above the inframammary fold.

The degrees of ptosis are usually classified as follows:

- *First degree (mild ptosis):* The nipple lies level with the inframammary fold.

- *Second degree (moderate ptosis):* The nipple droops below the inframammary fold but is still higher than the lowest portion of the breast.

- *Third degree (severe ptosis):* The nipple droops below the inframammary fold, may point downward, and is below the lowest part of the breast.

- *Pseudoptosis:* The nipple lies above the level of the inframammary fold, but most of the breast tissue falls below the fold.

Whether your ptosis is mild, moderate, or severe, you may want to consider a breast lift. This procedure can produce remarkable results regardless of the degree of sagging. You should note that breast lifts involve a variety of incisions that leave visible scars on the breasts. Some surgeons, however, specialize in performing breast lifts that leave minimal scarring. If you would like to minimize scarring, you may want to consider this possibility.

You also should be aware that when a significant amount of excess skin is removed from your breasts, it also may reduce the overall size of your breasts. Following a breast lift, you may find that you will need a smaller bra cup size. In some cases, however, if you have an abundance of extra tissue on the sides of your chest, that tissue may be folded into the breast to add more fullness.

Types of Breast Lifts

Several techniques can be used to perform a breast lift. Your surgeon will determine the best type of breast lift for you depending on the degree of sagging, your breast size, and the location and size of the nipple and areola.

Wise Pattern Breast Lift

When sagging is severe, as it often is after massive weight loss, a Wise pattern breast lift may be recommended. This technique also may be referred to as an *anchor breast lift* or an *inverted T breast lift* due to the shape of the scars it leaves on the breast. This procedure can remove significant

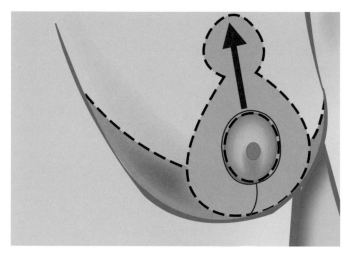

Wise pattern (anchor) breast lift. Skin shown within the dotted lines is removed. Red line shows scar.

amounts of excess skin from severely droopy breasts. A Wise pattern breast lift typically involves three incisions: a horizontal incision across the inframammary fold, a vertical incision from the nipple down to the inframammary fold, and an incision around the periphery of the areola. In some cases, the horizontal incision can be extended toward your back or underarm to remove excess tissue in those areas.

Vertical Breast Lift

A vertical breast lift involves a vertical incision from the areola to the inframammary fold and an incision around the areola, but no horizontal incision. This approach may be referred to as a

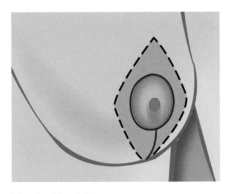

Vertical incision

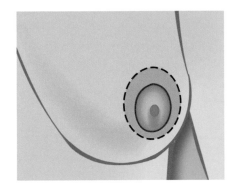

Doughnut incision

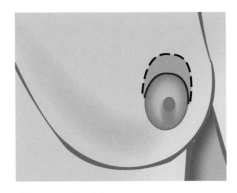

Crescent incision

lollipop breast lift because of the shape of the scar it leaves. Often recommended if you have mild to moderate sagging, a vertical breast lift also may be performed after massive weight loss in some cases.

Doughnut and Crescent Breast Lifts

If you have smaller breasts and minimal sagging, your surgeon may recommend a *doughnut breast lift* or *crescent breast lift*. These two techniques involve either a semi-circular or circular incision around the areola. There are no vertical or horizontal incisions. Only a small amount of excess skin can be removed with these techniques, and the amount of lift that can be achieved is minimal. These limited techniques usually aren't adequate if you have experienced massive weight loss.

Your Breast Lift Procedure

The amount of time required for a breast lift procedure can range from about one and a half hours to three and a half hours. Depending on the type of breast lift you're having, your surgeon will make the appropriate incisions on the breast. These incisions may include some combination of the following: a horizontal incision along the inframammary fold, a vertical incision from the areola to the inframammary fold, and an incision around the periphery of the areola.

Once the appropriate incisions have been made, excess skin will be removed. Next, your surgeon will lift the breast tissue and the nipple/areola complex from its droopy location to a more youthful position on the breast. If you also are having the nipple/areola complex reduced in size, it is typically performed at this time by trimming away the excess areola tissue. The remaining skin is draped around the breast tissue and pulled tight to provide support and create a more pleasing appearance.

At this point, your surgeon will begin closing the incisions with sutures. Drains may be inserted on each side to prevent fluid from building up following your surgery. In many cases, you will be placed in a binder or support bra to reduce post-operative swelling and to improve support.

Breast Lift with Augmentation

In some cases, a breast lift alone may not give you the volume and fullness you would like to achieve. This can occur if you don't have enough breast tissue to create the contours you want. When this is the case, you may want to consider breast augmentation in addition to a breast lift.

Breast augmentation is a surgical procedure that increases the size of your breasts by placing implants into the breasts. When combined with a breast lift, augmentation can dramatically reshape breasts that have lost their firmness. In most cases, this combined procedure produces a more attractive silhouette and better overall body proportions.

Depending on your unique physical characteristics and your goals, augmentation may be performed at the same time as a breast lift or may be staged. However, if you have a large amount of excess skin or a very long breast, you may experience premature sagging of the breast if an implant is placed at the same time as a lift. When the procedures are being staged, the breast lift is typically performed first, with augmentation taking place in a follow-up procedure.

One of the benefits of having augmentation in addition to a lift is that your incisions may be less extensive than if you were having a lift alone. Since the implant will add volume to the breast, it means that less skin may need to be removed. If you choose to have augmentation in addition to a breast lift, you will have several choices to make regarding the breast implants, which come in a wide variety of sizes, shapes, and textures. Some women choose autologous implants, meaning their own body tissue (fat) is used rather than implants.

Types of Implants

All breast implants have an outer shell made of silicone *elastomer* (a rubberlike substance), but they can be filled with either sterile saline or silicone gel. There are benefits and drawbacks associated with each of these types. Your surgeon can help you understand the differences between the two, but ultimately, the decision is yours.

Saline

Saline breast implants are filled with a sterile saline solution that is similar to fluids normally found in the body. If a saline implant ruptures or leaks, the fluid is simply absorbed by the body and

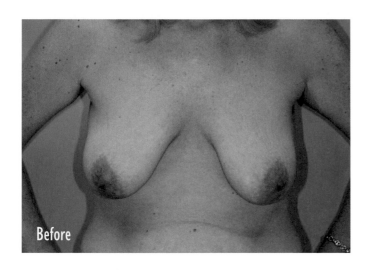

Before

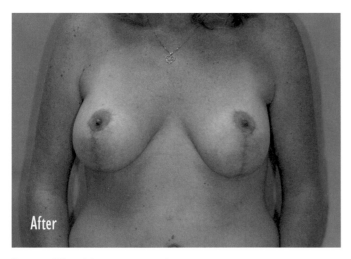

After

Breast lift with augmentation

flushed out during urination. For many years, saline implants were the only type of implant available to most women.

Saline implants are often prefilled to a certain size prior to surgery. Other variations of saline implants are filled during surgery to the size you and your surgeon have agreed upon. A few varieties also allow for minor adjustments in terms of volume and size for a short period of time following your procedure.

Silicone Gel

Silicone gel implants have a silicone elastomer shell that is filled with silicone gel. Many surgeons and women think silicone gel implants look and feel more natural than saline implants. That may explain why silicone gel implants are the most popular type of implant used outside of the United States. In the United States, however, silicone gel implants were not approved by the Food and Drug Administration (FDA) until 2006.

You may recall that in the 1990s, there was some controversy surrounding the safety of silicone gel implants. When leakage from a silicone gel implant occurs, it may be difficult for you or your surgeon to detect, and the silicone remains in the body rather than being flushed out. Concerns arose about a possible link between silicone gel implants that had ruptured or leaked and connective tissue diseases or cancer.

For years, the FDA restricted the use of silicone gel implants while large-scale studies were being performed to assess their safety. These clinical trials showed no evidence that silicone gel breast implants are associated with connective tissue disease or with cancer. Based on this evidence, the FDA approved the use of silicone gel breast implants in all women over the age of twenty-two.

Because it's difficult to tell if a silicone gel implant has ruptured, the FDA recommends periodic MRI scans to help detect any leaks. The FDA guidelines suggest a first MRI three years after your procedure and then every other year after that. You should be aware that your insurance may not cover these MRI scans.

Shapes of Implants

Originally, breast implants were only available in a round shape. Due to technical innovations, implants now come in both a round shape and an anatomical shape that is designed to create a more natural-shaped breast. Both of these shapes can produce excellent results. To determine which is best for you, consult with your surgeon.

Round

Whether you choose saline or silicone gel implants, the most popular shape used is round. Round implants typically provide greater fullness in the upper portion of the breast than would occur naturally. One of the biggest advantages of round implants is that if they rotate within the breast, there is no noticeable change.

Anatomical

Anatomical implants are designed to be fuller at the bottom than at the top, much like the shape of a natural breast. Also called *teardrop, contoured,* or *shaped* implants, anatomical implants were introduced to produce a more natural-looking breast. However, there is some debate in the medical community as to whether or not anatomical implants maintain their unique shape after being implanted in the body.

Although a rare occurrence, anatomical implants can rotate within the breast just as round implants can rotate. However, with anatomical implants, any rotation can cause a visible change in the shape of the breast. To minimize the risk of rotation, anatomical implants come with a textured outer shell that is designed to help keep the implants in place.

In addition, when silicone gel is used in anatomical implants, there is less likelihood of movement than with contoured saline implants. When rotation occurs, your surgeon may be able to shift the implant back into place manually. In very rare instances, minor surgery may be required to correct the problem.

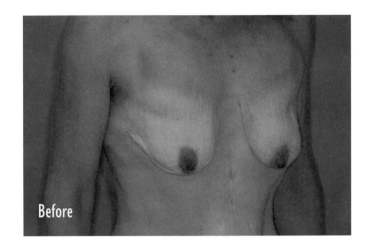

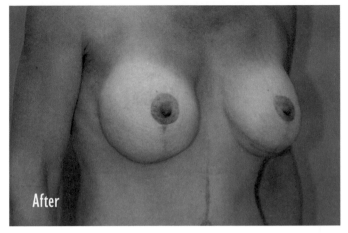

Breast lift with augmentation

Textures of Implants

The outer shell of the breast implant is available in two styles: smooth or textured. Both styles have advantages and disadvantages. Your surgeon will help you decide which texture is best for your needs.

Smooth

The most commonly used breast implants have a smooth outer shell. This smooth surface reduces the chances of developing certain problems associated with breast implants, such as visible rippling or wrinkling. Smooth implants are more likely to shift slightly within the breast; however, when smooth implants are round in shape, this typically doesn't produce any visible changes in the shape of the breast.

Textured

Textured implants have a rough outer shell that is designed to prevent the implants from shifting within the breast. Another reason that textured implants were introduced is that they may help prevent a complication associated with breast implant surgery called *capsular contracture*. (See the section on Risks Specific to Breast Aumentation Procedures in this chapter for more information on capsular contracture.) On the downside, textured implants have a greater tendency of developing visible wrinkling or rippling on the surface of the skin.

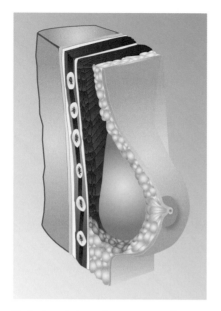

Subglandular placement of implant

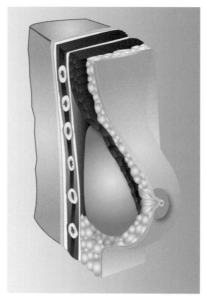

Submuscular placement of implant

Placement of Implants

Implants can be placed within the breasts in one of two positions. Implants may be placed partially below the pectoral muscle—*submuscular* placement—or on top of the pectoral muscle but below the breast tissue—*subglandular* placement.

Submuscular

With submuscular placement, the upper portion of the implant is positioned below the pectoral muscle, but the lower portion of the implant sits under the breast tissue. For a variety of reasons, most surgeons recommend submuscular placement. For instance, implants placed submuscularly are less likely to develop capsular contracture, one of the most common complications associated with breast implants.

In addition, when implants are positioned below the pectoral muscle, it reduces the occurrence of rippling and minimizes the risk of feeling or seeing the edges of the implant under the skin. Submuscular placement also causes less interference with future mammograms. Disadvantages associated with this method include a higher degree of post-operative discomfort and a slightly longer recovery period.

Subglandular

With subglandular placement, implants are placed below the breast tissue but on top of the chest muscle. Although subglandular placement isn't used as commonly as submuscular placement, it does have a few advantages. This method offers a quicker recovery time and less post-operative pain. On the downside, you may be at increased risk for capsular contracture, and you're more

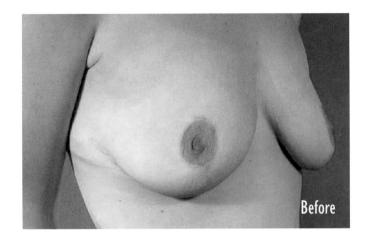

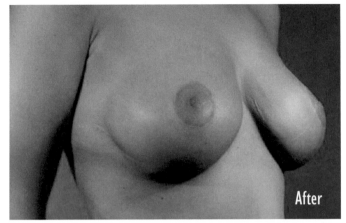

Breast lift with augmentation

likely to be able to feel or see the edges of the implant beneath the skin.

Size of Implants

Implants come in a wide range of sizes and are usually measured in cubic centimeters (cc). What's a cubic centimeter? It's a unit of measure that is typically used for volumes of fluid. Implant sizes can range from about 125 cc to more than 800 cc. To give you a point of reference, 30 cc is the equivalent of approximately 1 fluid ounce.

How do you choose which size is right for you? Unfortunately, selecting an implant size isn't easy, and there's no sure-fire method for zeroing in on the best size for you. You may think that all you have to do is tell your surgeon that you want

to be a C-cup or a B-cup. But this isn't very helpful because bra cup sizes aren't standardized among bra manufacturers and may actually differ from style to style from the same maker.

Possibly the best way to communicate your goals in terms of size is with photos. You can take images you find in magazines with you to your consultation. Many plastic surgeons also post their before-and-after photo galleries on the Internet. If you see results that are close to what you hope to achieve, you may want to print out a copy of the images you see on screen.

Of course, it's always a good idea to view your own surgeon's before-and-after photo gallery. Even if you don't find results that match your goals, you can still effectively communicate your desires by commenting on the images you see. For instance, simply saying that what you see in an image is "too big" or "too small" can give your surgeon an idea of what you hope to accomplish.

You may have heard that "trying on" breast implants in your bra is a good way to determine which size you should get. When you need a breast lift as well as augmentation, this approach will give you a good idea of your new size but not necessarily your new breast shape. That's because the shape of your breasts will change once your sagging skin is removed.

Your surgeon also will provide you with recommendations for size based on your physique and the amount of existing breast tissue you have. Of course, it's up to you to make the final decision on the size you would like your breasts to be.

Your Breast Lift with Augmentation Procedure

When augmentation is performed at the same time as a breast lift, it can take approximately two to four hours. Augmentation typically only takes one to two hours when performed as a follow-up procedure to a breast lift. When it's performed in a follow-up procedure, your surgeon will begin your augmentation procedure by re-opening a portion of the incisions made for the breast lift. After the incisions have been made, a "pocket" will be created within the breast. This pocket is where the implant will be placed and can be located either below the pectoral muscle or above it. Your surgeon will then insert the implant into the pocket.

The implant may be inserted prefilled, or it may be filled to a predetermined volume at this time during the procedure. When an implant is filled during surgery, small adjustments in volume may be made to create an optimal shape. Once the desired contours have been achieved, your surgeon will close the incisions using absorbable or nonabsorbable sutures. At the end of your procedure, you may be placed in an elastic binder or support bra.

Breast Reduction

If you feel that your breasts are too large, even after massive weight loss, you may be a candidate for a breast reduction. This surgical procedure typically involves the removal of excess fat, glandular breast tissue, and skin to reduce breast size to a more comfortable level.

Breast reduction is often performed if you are experiencing problems due to the weight of your breasts. For instance, large, heavy breasts commonly cause back and neck pain and may lead to poor posture. They also may leave you with skin irritations beneath the breasts. And when you wear a bra, you may experience deep gouging where the bra digs into your skin. A breast reduction can provide relief from these conditions by reducing the size and weight of your breasts.

Breast reduction may be covered by insurance if it is deemed to be medically necessary. Documentation showing that you suffer from problems associated with large breasts will be required if you plan to seek payment from your insurance company. In addition, insurance companies typically only cover reduction when a large portion of breast tissue is removed. Before scheduling your procedure, it's a good idea to contact your insurance company to find out exactly what their requirements are for breast reduction coverage.

Types of Breast Reduction

In general, the incisions used to perform a breast reduction are similar to those used to perform a breast lift. As a rule of thumb, the technique chosen depends on the composition of your breasts and the amount of reduction you desire.

Wise Pattern Breast Reduction

This approach involves the same incisions described for a Wise pattern breast lift. The Wise pattern is the most commonly used breast reduction technique, and it allows for the largest amount of breast tissue to be removed. In addition, with this procedure, the nipple and areola can be repositioned to a higher location on the breast mound, and your breasts can be contoured to a more pleasing shape.

Vertical Incision Breast Reduction

Depending on your needs, your surgeon may recommend a vertical incision breast reduction, which involves the same incisions used for a vertical, or lollipop breast lift. This approach results in less visible scarring on the breasts but may not be appropriate for removing large amounts of breast tissue. It is more likely to be suggested if you have only mild to moderate amounts of tissue to be removed. With this technique, the skin may bunch together where the incision meets the inframammary fold. In time, this bunching may resolve on its own, or in some cases, it may require a minor follow-up procedure, usually performed in the office under local anesthesia.

Limited Scar Breast Reduction

If the amount of tissue to be removed is minimal, a small incision around the nipple may be all that's necessary. This approach typically results in only a small change in breast size. For this reason, it isn't commonly recommended for breast reduction after massive weight loss.

Free Nipple Graft

In rare cases, extremely large breasts that need a very high volume of tissue reduction may require a method called *free nipple graft*. With this technique, the nipple and areola are completely detached from the underlying tissues of the breast and then reattached to a new position on the breast mound. With this method, there are certain

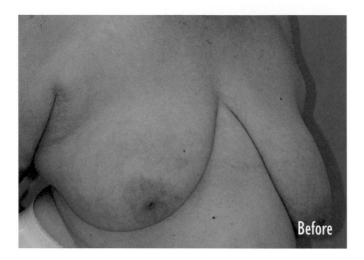

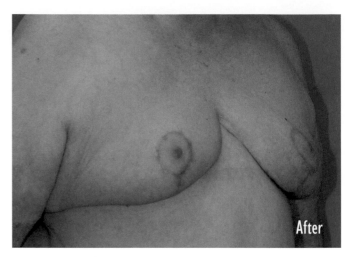

Breast reduction

disadvantages, including a loss of sensation in the nipple, the inability to breast-feed, and a lightening in color of the nipple and areola.

Your Breast Reduction Procedure

Breast reduction operations usually take approximately two to four hours. Your procedure will begin with the surgeon making incisions on one of your breasts. The surgeon will lift the skin away from the underlying breast tissue and remove tissue until the desired size is achieved. Minor liposuction also may be performed at the side of the breast or near the underarm to remove fat and to provide better contouring. Excised breast tissue is typically weighed as a way to maintain proper symmetry. In general, excised tissue is not

disposed of. Instead, it is sent to a pathology lab to check for any abnormal changes.

Once the breast has been reduced, any excess skin will be removed, and your nipple and areola will be moved to a higher position on the breast. Unless a free nipple transfer is being performed, the nipple and areola remain attached to the underlying tissue as it is moved. If necessary, your surgeon also will reduce the size of your areola by trimming away the excess.

Your surgeon will close the incisions using layers of sutures. Permanent sutures placed in the deep tissue provide additional support to help hold the breast in its new position on the chest wall. On the skin's surface, Steri-Strips or tissue

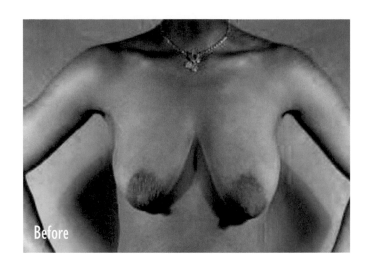
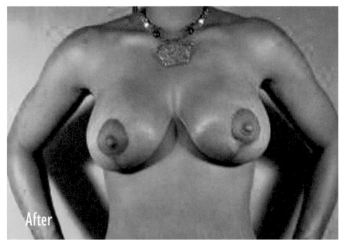

Breast lift with augmentation

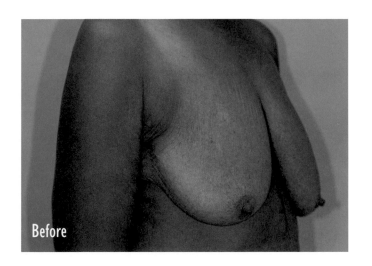
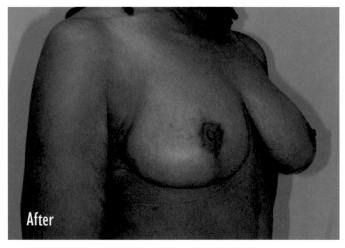

Breast lift with autologous augmentation

glue may be used. A drain may be placed into the surgical area.

At this point, your surgeon will repeat the procedure on your other breast. Before the incisions on your second breast are closed, your upper body will be shifted into an upright position so your surgeon can judge the size and symmetry of your breasts. If your breasts appear out of balance, the second breast can be fine-tuned until it matches your other breast more closely.

When your surgeon is satisfied with the outcome, a drain may be placed in the second breast, and the incisions will be closed. Gauze dressings are typically applied to the incisions, and your chest will be wrapped in snug-fitting bandages.

After Your Breast Procedure

After breast surgery, you will either go home the same day or spend one night in the hospital. Following your breast procedure, you can expect to experience mild to moderate pain, which can be controlled with the pain medications prescribed by your surgeon. Your breasts will look swollen and may feel tight and firm. This swelling may increase in the first few days after surgery before beginning to subside.

Recovering from Your Breast Procedure

Your surgeon will give you specific post-operative instructions to help minimize your discomfort and speed your recovery. These instructions may include details on sleeping positions, wearing a support bra, emptying any drains, personal hygiene, restricting activities, and returning to work.

After breast surgery, you will be advised to try to sleep on your back for at least one week. However, if you absolutely cannot get any sleep in this position, you may be allowed to sleep on your side. To help reduce swelling, prop up your upper body by placing a couple of pillows behind you while you are in bed.

With breast reduction surgery, your chest will typically be wrapped in bandages. These bandages will be replaced within a few days after your surgery and then will remain in place until your drains are removed. After that, you will be asked to wear a surgical bra day and night for about two to three weeks.

For a breast lift or a breast lift with augmentation, you'll be instructed to wear a support bra or sports bra at all times for about two to three weeks. After that, you can usually wear any bra that feels comfortable during the day, although underwire bras are not advised.

If you have any drains, which are commonly used for breast reduction surgery, you will be given instructions on how to empty them. Typically, it is okay to shower with the drains still in place as long as you don't soak the drain sites. Showering is usually allowed once your gauze dressings have been removed, usually within a few days after your procedure.

After a breast lift or a lift with augmentation, you will need to avoid aerobic activities for at least three weeks and heavy lifting for about two weeks. With breast reduction procedures, you typically need to wait about six weeks to resume strenuous activities. In most cases, you can return to work in about one to two weeks.

Risks of Breast Procedures

Potential complications that can occur with a breast lift or breast reduction procedure include the following.

- *Shooting or burning pains:* Temporary burning, tingling, or shooting pains are associated with the healing and regeneration of sensory nerves.

- *Asymmetry:* At first, your breasts may not appear to be symmetrical. This may be due to the fact that each breast heals independently as you recover. For example, swelling may be more noticeable in one breast. Once you've

completely healed, symmetry usually returns.

- *Change in nipple sensation:* One or both of your nipples may feel temporarily numb or extremely sensitive to touch.

- *Breast hardness:* Areas of the breast may feel hard due to post-surgical scarring within the breast.

- *Bottoming out:* With reduction surgery, the lower half of the breast skin may stretch, causing the breast tissue to droop below the level of the nipple. This condition may be corrected with a minor revision procedure.

- *Interference with breast-feeding:* With breast reduction, your ability to breast-feed may be impaired.

- *Continued pain:* Breast reduction may not effectively relieve pre-existing back or neck pain.

Risks Specific to Breast Augmentation Procedures

When breast augmentation is performed in addition to a breast lift, there are additional risks, such as the following.

- *Capsular contracture:* The most common complication following the insertion of breast implants is capsular contracture. When implants are placed in the body, a

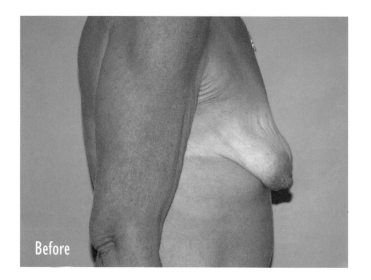

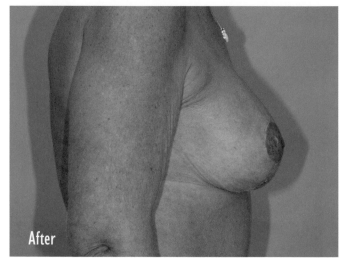

Breast lift with augmentation

layer of scar tissue normally forms around the implant. In some cases, this scar tissue contracts and squeezes the implant. This can lead to excessive firmness and may change the shape of the breast or cause pain. Symptoms can range from mild to severe with the most severe cases requiring follow-up surgery.

■ *Rupture/Deflation/Leakage:* Implants may leak, rupture, or deflate if the outer shell is compromised. Studies show that saline implants leak at a rate of 1 to 2 percent over many years. If an implant ruptures or deflates, it will need to be surgically replaced. Implant manufacturers typically offer warranties on breast implants, and

the cost of a new implant may be covered.

■ *Hematoma:* Although rare, blood may pool around the implant. This is known as a hematoma, which can cause pain and swelling and may contribute to capsular contracture. Most hematomas are small and will resolve on their own. More severe cases may require treatment in your surgeon's office.

■ *Implant Visibility/Palpability:* More commonly with subglandular placement, you may be able to see or feel the edges of the implant under the skin.

- *Wrinkling:* With saline implants, you may have surface irregularities, such as wrinkling.

- *Capsule Calcification:* Calcium deposits may occur in the scar capsule that forms around the implant. These calcium deposits may interfere with mammography.

- *Interference with Mammography:* Breast implants may interfere with traditional mammography. However, a special viewing method called the Eklund technique can be used to improve the effectiveness of mammography in women with implants. Be sure to inform the technician that you have breast implants so this special technique can be used.

- *Exposure/Extrusion of Implant:* In very rare cases, the skin can erode, allowing the implant to become visible through the skin.

- *Synmastia:* A very unusual occurrence, synmastia causes the skin between the two breasts to pull away from the breastbone, reducing or eliminating the appearance of cleavage. If this unusual complication develops, it will require additional surgery.

Breast Surgery Facts

- Length of Surgery: 1 to 4 hours
- Type of Anesthesia: General or local with sedation
- Hospital Stay: 1 to 2 days
- Pain Level: Mild to moderate
- Drains: For breast reduction, usually removed in 1 to 3 weeks
- Compression Garment: Support bra for at least 2 weeks
- Visible Sutures: Usually only around the areola, removed in 5 to 7 days in office
- Activity Restrictions: No strenuous activity or heavy lifting for 2 to 6 weeks
- Return to Work: 1 to 2 weeks
- Final Outcome: 6 to 12 months

How Long Will Breast Procedures Last?

Breast lifts permanently remove excess skin, and the results are typically long-lasting. However, if you are prone to loose skin, sagging may return over time. With breast reduction procedures, the size of your breasts is permanently reduced.

Similarly, however, sagging may occur as you age, altering the youthful contours achieved with your surgery. If you choose breast implants, a larger and heavier implant will likely cause the breast to sag more with time.

Breast implants are designed to be long-lasting, and as long as you aren't experiencing any problems, you don't need to replace them. However, implants are not considered lifetime devices and may require removal or replacement at some point during your lifetime. Rest assured that if this occurs, implant manufacturers offer lifetime product-replacement warranties. However, the costs of surgery associated with removal or replacement may not be covered.

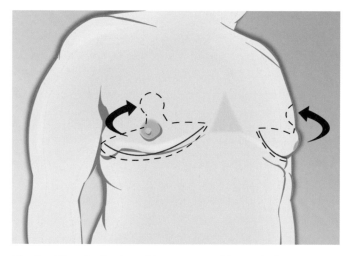

Dotted line indicates skin removed in male breast reduction. Red line shows scar.

Be aware that weight fluctuations or pregnancy following any type of breast surgery can dramatically alter the results of your procedure. For instance, it can cause breasts that have been lifted to stretch and sag. And breasts that have been surgically reduced in size once again may enlarge during pregnancy or due to weight gain. In most cases, it is recommended to maintain a stable weight and to wait until after you've finished bearing children to have breast surgery.

Male Breast Reduction

If you're a man who feels awkward or embarrassed by enlarged breasts or sagging on your chest, you may want to consider male breast reduction. When you're obese, it's very common to experience breast enlargement, a medical condition known as *gynecomastia*. And when you lose a large amount of weight, your chest area may start to look saggy. Both of these conditions can be treated with plastic surgery.

Male breast reduction enhances the contours of the chest area by removing excess skin, fat, and glandular tissue. It also can improve the size and position of your areolas if they have been stretched out due to severe gynecomastia or sagging. Be aware that some procedures to reshape the male chest involve incisions that will result in visible scarring.

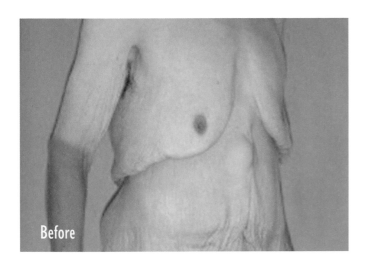
Before

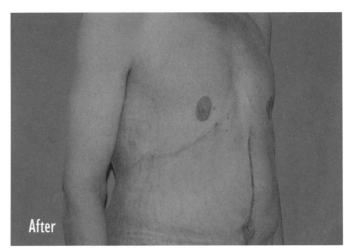
After

Male breast reduction

Your Male Breast Reduction Procedure

Male breast reduction surgery usually takes about two to three hours. In many cases, liposuction is the first step in male chest contouring. In fact, if excess fatty tissue is the primary cause of your enlarged breasts, liposuction may be the only technique necessary.

To remove excess skin or breast tissue, your surgeon will make an incision on the chest. The incisions used will depend on your particular situation but commonly include a horizontal incision along the crease of the breast. Depending on the amount and location of excess skin and tissue, this incision may extend to your side. A circular incision around the areola will be necessary if the nipple and areola need to be moved into a higher position.

Once the incisions have been made, glandular tissue and excess skin will be excised. If necessary, the nipple and areola will be repositioned to a more natural location on the chest. The nipple and areola may remain attached to the underlying tissues when moved, or the nipple and areola may be removed completely and replaced as a skin graft.

When the optimal contours have been achieved, your surgeon will insert a drain into each side of the chest and will close the incisions with layers of sutures. Gauze dressings will be placed on your incisions, and a compression garment will be placed around your chest.

After Your Male Breast Reduction Procedure

You will usually go home the same day after your male breast reduction procedure. Following male chest contouring, you can expect to experience mild pain that can be controlled with either prescription pain medication or over-the-counter pain relievers. Swelling may be pronounced at first but may be mostly resolved after about four to six weeks. By wearing the compression garment as instructed, you can help reduce swelling. Expect to return to work in about one to two weeks. Resuming strenuous activities, however, may take four to six weeks.

11

Arm and Upper Body Procedures

Are you embarrassed to wear short-sleeved shirts because a large amount of skin droops from your underarms? Is it hard to find shirts that fit due to that extra skin? Unfortunately, no amount of exercising or strength training will get rid of those flaps of skin that drape from your elbow to your underarm. If you're bothered by the way your arms look, you may be a candidate for an arm lift. This surgical procedure, which also is called *brachioplasty,* improves the shape and tone of your arms. Arm lifts are becoming more and more popular following massive weight loss, with nearly 15,000 procedures performed each year.

Arm Lift

An arm lift is a surgical procedure that redefines the contours of your arms from the elbow to the underarm. This procedure permanently removes drooping skin that may be due to massive weight loss, the natural aging process, or simple heredity. In some cases, liposuction also may be performed to remove pockets of fat and fine-tune the contours of your arms.

It's important to understand that arm lifts leave visible scars that usually extend from the elbow to the underarm. In this case, the procedure is known as a *standard brachioplasty.* If you have additional excess skin in the underarm area, you may require what's called an *extended brachioplasty,* in which the incision extends beyond the underarm to the side of the chest.

For minor amounts of extra tissue that are confined to the uppermost part of the arm, a *short-scar brachioplasty* may be performed, in which the incision begins above the elbow. However, following massive weight loss, a short-scar brachioplasty typically can't remove an adequate amount of excess tissue to provide a satisfactory result.

Arm lifts can be performed alone but are often done in combination with other procedures, such as breast lifts or upper body lifts, which will be discussed in greater detail later in this chapter.

Your Arm Lift Procedure

When performed alone, an arm lift typically takes about two hours. The procedure begins with an incision along the inner arm or the back of the arm. Depending on the amount of excess tissue to be removed, the incision may extend past the elbow to the forearm or past the underarm to the side of the chest. In these cases, a Z-shaped incision may be used at the elbow or underarm.

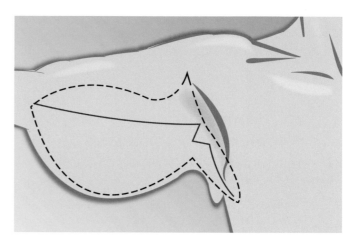

Extended arm lift incision

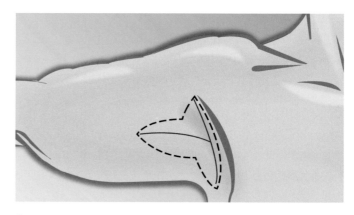

Short-incision arm lift incision

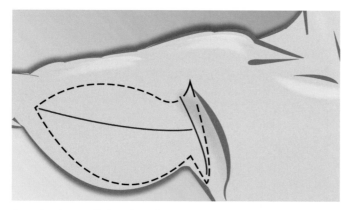

Standard arm lift incision. Skin shown within the dotted lines is removed. Red line shows scar.

This can prevent the resulting scar from tightening and constricting movement.

After the incision has been made, liposuction may be performed to remove fat deposits. Then excess skin and tissue are removed until satisfactory contours are achieved. A surgical drain may be placed in the arm, and the incision is closed using layers of sutures. The process is repeated on the other arm, with great care taken to maintain symmetry in the size of your arms.

After Your Arm Lift Procedure

A hospital stay usually isn't necessary after an arm lift if that's the only procedure being performed. In most cases, you'll go home the same day. Typically, you'll be sent home with drains near the surgical site and compression garments on your upper arms. Following an arm lift, pain is often described as mild to moderate and can be controlled with prescription pain medications or over-the-counter pain relievers.

Recovering from Your Arm Lift Procedure

Arm lifts are usually associated with a rapid and relatively easy recovery. As your arms heal, you'll be advised to follow your doctor's post-operative instructions. For instance, you'll be informed how and when to empty your drains. In addition, you may be asked to wear compression garments at some point during your recovery. To reduce swelling, keep your arms propped up on a couple of pillows while you're lying in bed or sitting in a chair.

Typically, following an arm lift, you'll be able to use your arms for your normal daily activities, such as brushing your teeth, eating, and getting dressed. However, you will be advised to move

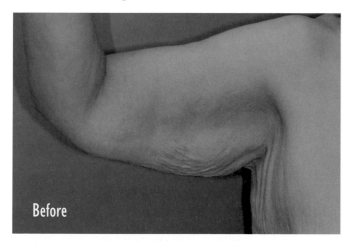

Before

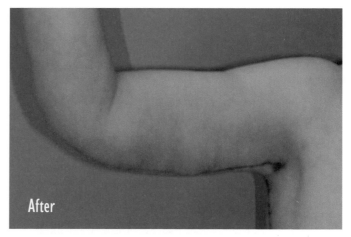

After

Arm lift

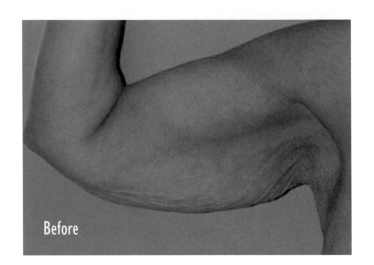
Before

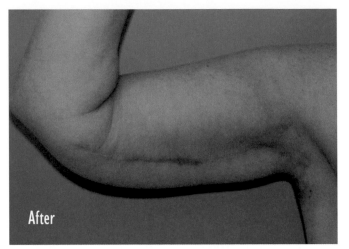
After

Arm lift

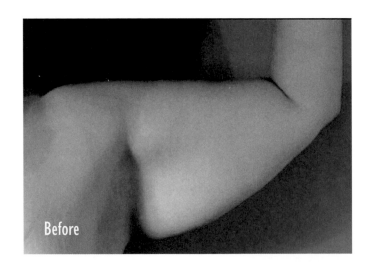
Before

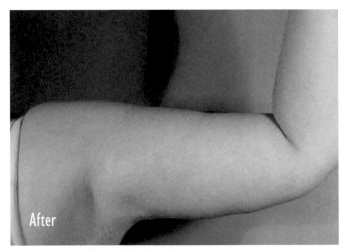
After

Arm lift

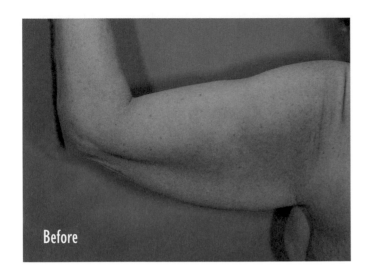

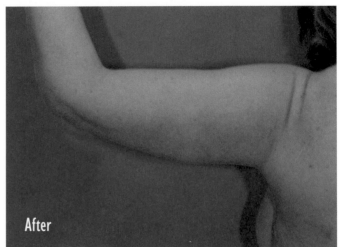

Arm lift

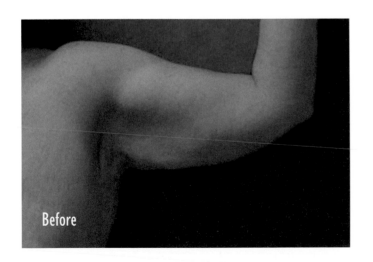

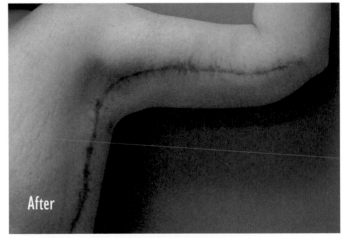

Arm lift with extension on to side of chest

Arm and Upper Body Procedures

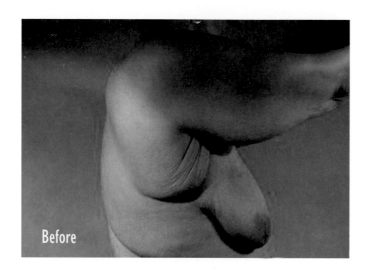

Before

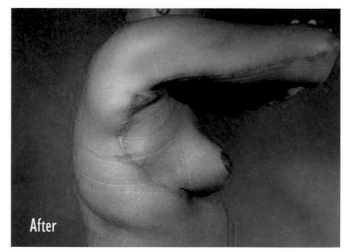

After

Upper torsoplasty. This procedure corrects sagging breasts and excess skin on the arms and sides of the chest.

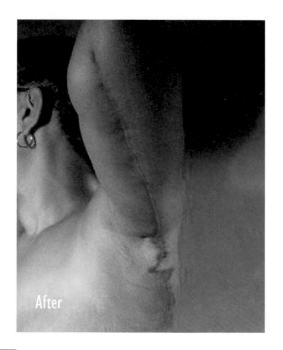

After

your arms carefully and to be gentle with your arm movements for about three to four weeks. Heavy lifting should be avoided for about six weeks, but you may be able to engage in other activities sooner than with most bariatric plastic surgery procedures. In fact, your surgeon may advise you to let pain be your guide. That means that if an activity causes pain, you should stop.

Risks of Arm Lifts

The general risks of surgery listed earlier also apply to arm lifts, which also are associated with the following specific risks.

- *Uneven skin contours:* In spite of your surgeon's best efforts, the skin on your arms may appear uneven, with slight depressions, rippling, or wrinkling.

- *Differences in size:* Your surgeon will make every effort to make your arms appear equal in size, but in most cases, there may be slight differences. You should realize that, usually, the two arms are not exactly the same size pre-operatively either.

- *Asymmetrical scars:* The scars on each arm heal independently and may not be completely symmetrical.

- *Interference with lymph system:* In rare cases, temporary interference with the lymph drainage system may occur. When this happens, it is usually minor and may require a compression stocking to be worn on the upper arm for a period of time.

How Long Will an Arm Lift Last?

Arm lifts, which permanently remove excess skin and fatty tissue from the upper arms, are generally considered to be long-lasting. Maintaining a stable weight and engaging in a physician-approved exercise routine can help you keep your arms looking as good as possible. However, since the skin on the upper arms is thin and delicate, it may be more prone to recurrent

Arm Lift Facts

- Length of Surgery: 2 to 4 hours
- Type of Anesthesia: General
- Hospital Stay: No
- Pain Level: Mild to moderate
- Drains: Yes, usually removed in 1 to 2 weeks
- Compression Garment: Sometimes, starting a few days after surgery
- Visible Sutures: Usually none to be removed
- Activity Restrictions: No strenuous activity or heavy lifting for 3 to 4 weeks
- Return to Work: 1 to 2 weeks
- Final Outcome: 6 to 12 months

laxity. In some cases, this may necessitate a minor revisionary procedure.

Upper Body Lift

Whether you're male or female, an upper body lift can remove excess skin and reshape the upper areas of the body. There is no standard guideline for which procedures are included for an upper body lift, also referred to as a torsoplasty; but this procedure may include any combination of your arms, breasts, chest, back, or sides. For instance, depending on your needs and your surgeon's preferred surgical technique, an upper body lift may involve only an arm lift and a breast lift. In other cases, it also may include the removal of loose skin from your back and the sides of your chest.

Depending on the number of areas treated, your upper body may undergo a complete transformation. Instead of loose, hanging skin, you will notice a more toned and attractive shape. For instance, if you're a woman, your breasts can be restored to a more youthful appearance, and your arms will look more slender. Or, if you're a man, your chest will have a more masculine shape, and your back may be rid of unsightly folds. When upper body procedures are combined, you can typically expect more balanced overall proportions.

As mentioned earlier, an upper body lift can involve a variety of procedures. It also may be performed using a number of different surgical techniques. The method your surgeon chooses depends on your individual needs as well as his or her personal preference. No matter which techniques your surgeon employs, you should achieve more satisfactory contours.

Your Upper Body Lift Procedure

Depending on the number of upper body areas targeted, an upper body lift can take four to six hours or sometimes even longer. The order in which your procedure is performed typically depends on

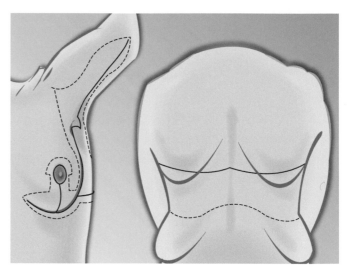

An upper body lift commonly includes excess skin removal from the upper back, sides, breasts, and arms. Skin shown within the dotted lines is removed. Red line shows scar.

your surgeon's personal preference. The procedure usually begins with either your back or your breasts or chest.

When the back is treated first, your body will be placed on its side. Your surgeon will begin by making a horizontal incision along the back in the area that would typically be hidden below a woman's bra strap. The incision may extend from the middle of the back to the side of the chest. Excess skin is removed, and liposuction may be performed to fine-tune the contours of the back. Then your body will be gently rolled onto the

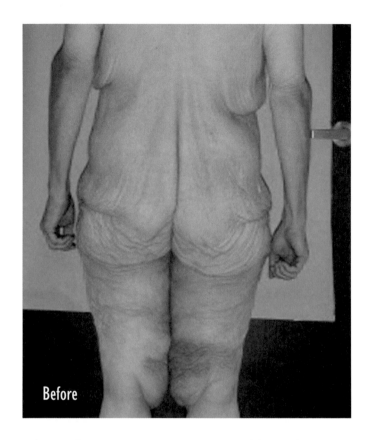

Before

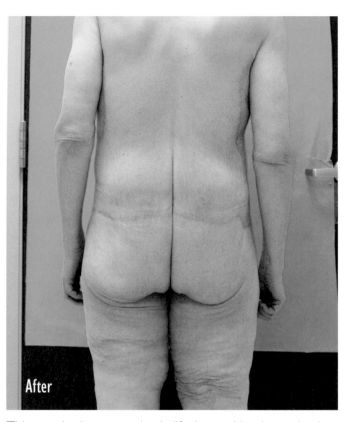

After

This man had an upper body lift along with a lower body lift, an inner thigh lift, and an arm lift.

other side so your surgeon can address the other side of your back.

Once your back has been contoured, you'll be rolled over, and your surgeon may continue with an arm lift. To do so, he or she will make incisions that extend from the side of the chest up to the underarm and down the inner sides or the backs of the arms. Once again, your surgeon will remove the loose skin and may perform minimal liposuction in the area to achieve the best shape.

The surgeon will then shift the focus to your chest. For a breast lift, a Wise pattern incision is commonly used, involving a circular incision around the nipple, a vertical incision from the nipple to the inframammary fold, and a horizontal incision along the inframammary fold. The incision made in the crease below the breast typically blends into the incisions that extend from the back.

Sagging skin is excised from the breasts, and the nipple is repositioned to a more youthful position on the breast mound. In some cases, breast implants also may be used to add fullness to your breasts. Your surgeon will carefully judge the shaping of your breasts to improve symmetry.

For male chest contouring, liposuction is typically performed before any skin is removed. Incisions on the male chest typically include a horizontal incision along the lower crease of the breast and may include a circular incision around the nipple if the nipple needs to be repositioned higher on the chest. The horizontal incision usually blends in with the incisions on your back.

A variation of the upper body lift procedure involves removing hanging skin from the back without using the horizontal incisions on the back. In this variation, your surgeon may extend the incision used for an arm lift beyond the underarm and vertically down the sides of the chest. In this manner, sagging back skin can be pulled laterally toward the side of the chest and trimmed off, resulting in smoother contours on the back and fewer visible scars.

Before completing your operation, your surgeon will place drains in the surgical areas to reduce the risk of fluid build-up. Your incisions will be closed using layers of sutures, and the surgical sites will be wrapped with gauze dressings

Upper Body Lift Facts

- Length of Surgery: 4 to 6 hours

- Type of Anesthesia: General

- Hospital Stay: 1 to 2 days

- Pain Level: Mild to moderate

- Drains: Yes, usually removed in 1 to 2 weeks

- Compression Garment: Sometimes, starting a few days after surgery

- Visible Sutures: Usually only around the areola, removed in 5 to 7 days in office. Skin glue also may be used requiring no suture removal and allowing you to shower or bathe immediately after surgery.

- Activity Restrictions: No strenuous activity or heavy lifting for 4 to 6 weeks

- Return to Work: 1 to 2 weeks

- Final Outcome: 6 to 12 months

to absorb any blood or fluid. Your breasts will likely be wrapped tightly in bandages to provide support.

After Your Upper Body Lift Procedure

After having combined upper body procedures, you may need to spend a day or two in the hospital. An IV will likely be attached to your arm or to the back of your hand in order to administer pain medication, antibiotics, and other fluids. Combined upper body procedures usually cause mild to moderate pain that can be well-controlled with pain medication.

To minimize pain while you are in the hospital, you also may be outfitted with a PCA device that allows you to administer pre-measured doses of pain medication as needed. You can expect the IV and the PCA device to be removed before you go home from the hospital.

During your hospital stay, the nursing staff will be in charge of emptying your drains and changing your dressings. They also will assist you with early walking. Prior to being discharged from the hospital, you will be instructed how to care for your drains and how to change your dressings.

Recovering from Your Upper Body Lift Procedure

You should expect recovery to take some time after an upper body lift because several areas of your body have been treated. Depending on your surgeon, you may be instructed to wear a vest-like compression garment or a support bra at all times for a few weeks. Your surgeon will let you know when you can switch to wearing a regular bra style.

If you have drains, you'll also be instructed to empty them and to record the amount of fluid that is collected in the bulbs. The drains will usually be removed in your surgeon's office in about one to two weeks. However, as long as there is fluid draining, the drains will need to remain in place.

As with most bariatric plastic surgery procedures, you will be instructed to avoid aerobic activities and heavy lifting for about four to six weeks. When your surgeon indicates that you can resume vigorous exercise, it's best to increase your activity levels gradually. Although your arms may be sore immediately following an upper body lift, you should be able to use them for routine daily activities. Just be sure to move your arms gently at first, elevate them according to your surgeon's directions, and avoid any activities that cause pain.

Staging or Combining Your Procedure?

When upper body procedures are combined, the results can be remarkable. You can go from having to wear loose-fitting shirts to accommodate or hide your hanging skin to having the confidence to dress in sleeveless and more form-fitting attire. You also may like the idea of a single recovery period after a combined procedure.

However, you should be aware that upper body lifts that target sagging skin on the back in addition to the breasts and the arms aren't very commonly performed in one operation. Most surgeons prefer to stage these procedures or only may address loose skin on the breasts and the arms but not on the back. Discuss these options with your surgeon so you can determine if a combined upper body lift is right for you.

Risks of Upper Body Lifts

In addition to the general risks of surgery discussed earlier, upper body lifts involve the same risks that are associated with arm lifts and breast surgery.

- *Shooting or burning pains:* Your breasts may experience temporary burning, tingling, or shooting pains as the sensory nerves heal.

- *Asymmetry:* You may notice asymmetry in the size of your breasts or your arms during the healing period, but this usually resolves once you're completely recovered. Note that slight differences in breast size are present in nearly all women before surgery and may be permanent.

- *Change in nipple sensation:* You may experience numbness or heightened sensitivity in one or both of your nipples.

- *Breast hardness:* Post-operative scarring can create areas of hardness within the breast.

- *Uneven skin contours:* You may notice rippling or wrinkling on your arms.

- *Asymmetrical scars:* Scars on the arms, breast, and back heal independently and may not be completely symmetrical.

- *Interference with lymph system:* During an arm lift, temporary interference with the lymph drainage system may occur, but this is rare. Treatment may include wearing a compression garment on the upper arm.

How Long Will an Upper Body Lift Last?

An upper body lift involves the permanent removal of hanging skin from the upper torso and the arms. Usually, the results are long-lasting, but there may be some recurrent skin laxity, especially on the arms. If the amount of skin looseness bothers you, you may want to opt for a secondary procedure to tighten the contours of your arms.

Of course, gaining and losing a major amount of weight can significantly alter the results you've achieved. Similarly, if you become pregnant following an upper body lift, your breasts may stretch and subsequently sag. Because of this, most surgeons will advise you to have an upper body lift once you've made the decision not to have any more children.

12

Face and Neck Procedures

After shedding a great deal of weight, you may feel healthier and younger than ever. In spite of these feelings, your face and neck may actually appear to have aged following weight loss. That's because the fullness of your face may have been replaced by drooping skin that makes you look older than you are. In general, the sagging that affects the face and neck after weight loss is far milder than the excess skin that hangs from the body. However, the unwanted changes to your face can't be easily hidden with clothing and may bother you. If you would like to improve your appearance, you may want to talk to your bariatric plastic surgeon about procedures that rejuvenate the face and neck.

Facelift

A facelift is a surgical procedure that restores a more refreshed and youthful appearance to the face and neck. Also called a *rhytidectomy,* a facelift typically addresses the lower two-thirds of the face in addition to the neck. This procedure tightens loose skin as well as the underlying muscles of the face and neck to achieve a more radiant, natural look. Wrinkles and creases in the facial skin also can be smoothed with a facelift.

Although there are a number of facelift techniques and procedures currently available, the SMAS facelift is the standard facelift technique used following massive weight loss. The SMAS refers to the *subcutaneous musculoaponeurotic system,* which is the layer of muscles that lie beneath the skin. With this facelift technique, the underlying SMAS is tightened to produce a smoother, more natural-looking facelift. Several decades ago, before the SMAS lifts were performed, only the skin was tightened; this approach resulted in a stretched, pulled appearance. Depending on your needs, your surgeon may recommend a

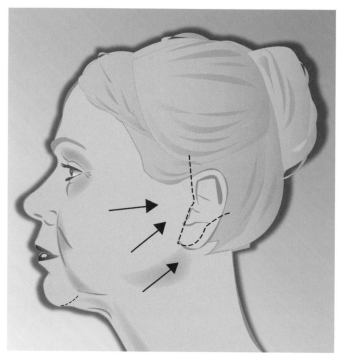

Incisions for a standard face lift. The dotted line shows the incision behind the ear.

Neck Lift

Also called a *cervicoplasty,* a neck lift addresses sagging skin on the neck. Although a neck lift can be performed alone, it is typically performed in combination with a facelift, especially if you're a weight loss patient. That's because a neck lift alone usually isn't adequate to remove the amount of excess skin that results from significant weight loss. A cervicoplasty only removes excess skin. If necessary, the underlying muscles within the neck, which are called plastysmal bands, also may be tightened. When the neck muscles are tightened, this is referred to as a *platysmaplasty.* Your surgeon may decide to perform both a cervicoplasty and a platysmaplasty to achieve the desired results.

Combining a Facelift with Other Procedures

To provide a more balanced and youthful appearance, you may want to consider additional facial procedures. For instance, you may benefit from upper and lower eyelid surgery *(blepharoplasty)* to reduce the appearance of heavy eyelids. A *browlift,* also called a *forehead lift,* also may be appealing to you if you would like to minimize a drooping brow. These procedures are commonly performed at the same time as a facelift.

variation of the SMAS facelift. For instance, if you have noticeable *nasolabial folds* or sagging fat pads under the cheeks, you may benefit from a procedure called an *extended SMAS facelift.* This procedure minimizes lines around the nose and mouth.

CHAPTER 12

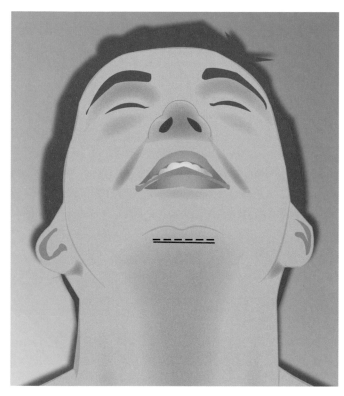

Dotted line indicates incision for male neck lift. Red line shows scar.

Your Facelift and Neck Lift Procedure

A combined facelift and neck lift procedure usually takes about two to four hours and often addresses the neck area first. Your surgeon will begin by making a small incision below the chin. Liposuction may be performed in the neck area to remove small deposits of fat. If necessary, the thin sheet of muscle covering the neck area will be tightened using sutures.

At this time, your surgeon may make the incisions for your facelift. The locations of these incisions vary but are often placed within the hairline at the temple, then extended downward in front of the ear, under the earlobe, and finally, behind the ear into the hairline. If you're a man, the incision locations may differ to avoid changes to the sideburns.

Once the incisions have been made, the skin is gently lifted away from the underlying fat and muscle. Your surgeon may fine-tune the distribution of fat below the skin either by performing liposuction or by performing fat grafts. Liposuction removes fat deposits, and fat grafts add fat to soften areas that appear hollow. If fat grafts are necessary, your surgeon may take fat from the neck or another part of the body and inject it into the cheeks or other areas of the face.

Next, the SMAS layer is tightened using sutures, the skin is redraped over the underlying tissues, and excess skin is trimmed away. Great care is used not to pull the skin too tight, and the incisions are closed without tension. Depending on your surgeon's personal preference, your incisions may be closed with absorbable or nonabsorbable sutures, staples, or some combination thereof.

Surgical drains may be placed at the sides of the face, and bulky gauze dressings are wrapped around the head and neck. Your surgeon also may place a compression garment that fits snugly around your neck and head.

After Your Facelift and Neck Lift Procedure

Following a facelift and neck lift, you may go home the same day, or you may be monitored overnight in the hospital or in an outpatient facility. You can expect your face to feel swollen and tight immediately after surgery. The bulky dressings used are designed to apply pressure to the surgical sites and to absorb any blood. After your facial procedure, you may not experience a great deal of pain. In fact, many facelift patients describe post-operative pain as mild and use nothing more than over-the-counter pain relievers to alleviate discomfort.

If you have drains, they may be removed the day after your procedure before you return home. In addition, the bulky gauze dressings may be replaced the day after your operation with light dressings.

Recovering from Your Facelift and Neck Lift Procedure

To speed healing and improve your comfort, be sure to follow your doctor's post-operative instructions. You may be asked to wear a compression garment that wraps around your head and neck at all times for the first week and at night for the second week following surgery.

To reduce swelling, apply ice packs, and keep your head elevated throughout the day and while you sleep at night. Place several pillows behind your back to keep your head above the level of your heart. Note that swelling often migrates downward to the neck area. This may create an unpleasant tightness in the neck area, but rest assured that this sensation decreases as time passes. Due to facial swelling, your eyelids also may feel tight at first.

Following facelift surgery, you also may notice some areas of lumpiness or firmness under the skin. This typically resolves within two to four months; however, gently massaging the hard areas may speed their resolution. Numbness also may be present but usually dissipates within a couple of months in the lower face, cheek, and neck areas. Forehead and scalp numbness may take up to a year to disappear.

Any visible sutures will be removed within a week, and any staples used are typically removed in one to two weeks. Once your sutures have been removed, you can begin wearing makeup again. You may have to wait about four to six weeks before you can dye your hair, so you may want to schedule a hair appointment right before your procedure.

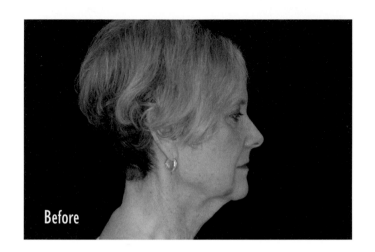

Before

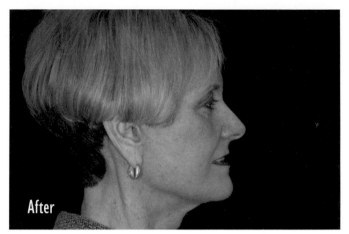

After

Facelift

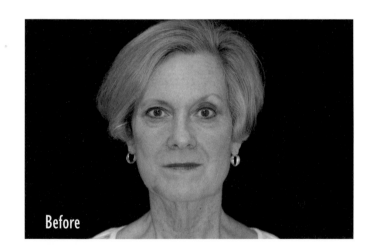

Before

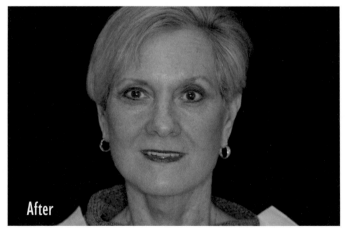

After

Facelift

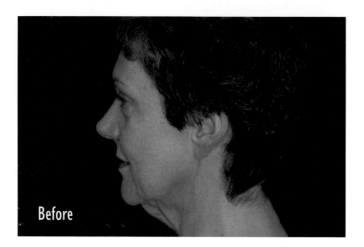

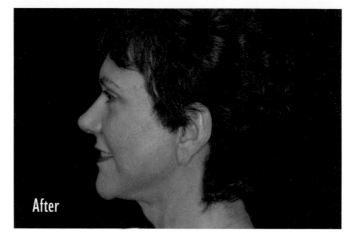

Facelift

Since the pain associated with facelifts is typically mild, you may begin feeling fairly normal within the first week. Even though you are feeling better, avoid strenuous activities and heavy lifting for at least three weeks. Engaging in aerobic activities sooner could lead to excessive bleeding or prolonged swelling. You may, however, return to light office work within about a week.

Risks of Facelifts and Neck Lifts

The general risks of surgery apply to procedures that target the face and neck. In addition, the following risks should be noted.

- *Hematoma:* When skin is pulled away from the underlying tissues, there is a chance that blood may pool under the skin. If a hematoma occurs in the neck area, it can lead to a life-threatening obstruction of the airway. The risk for hematoma is often cited as the main reason that plastic surgeons prefer to have facelift patients monitored overnight following surgery. This way, a hematoma can be treated immediately before it becomes a danger.

- *Nerve injury:* Although rare, it is possible for nerves to be injured during surgery. This may result in temporary weakness of one or both sides of the lower lip. It may take several months for symptoms to disappear completely.

- *Necrosis:* If skin is pulled too tight or if you're a smoker, there is an increased chance of skin death. Skin loss occurs most commonly behind the ear. This can prolong the healing period and may result in visible scarring.

- *Injury to deeper structures:* On rare occasions, underlying muscles or blood vessels may be injured.

- *Numbness:* Permanent numbness occurs rarely, but when it does, it usually involves the earlobes or the area in front of the ear.

- *Chronic pain:* Although discomfort is usually mild and short-lived following a facelift, it may become chronic in very rare cases.

- *Hair loss:* Hair along the incision lines within the scalp may be lost.

How Long Will a Facelift and Neck Lift Last?

It's hard to say exactly how long your facelift and neck lift will last, but in general, the results last about ten to twelve years. Your individual results will depend on a number of factors, including your skin quality. Often, the younger you are, the more elasticity your skin has, and the longer your results will last. As you age, however, your skin loses that ability to snap back when pulled, and you may notice recurring sagging sooner.

Skin Rejuvenation

When it comes to facial cosmetic surgery, a facelift can eliminate loose skin and tighten underlying tissues to give your face a smoother, more youthful contour; however, a facelift does not change the condition of the surface of your skin. You may have fine wrinkles or skin damage that you'd also like to eliminate. If so, you may want to consider skin rejuvenation treatments to enhance the appearance of your skin. Many of these treatments can be performed in your plastic surgeon's office and require no downtime. That's part of the reason that these procedures have become some of the most popular cosmetic treatments available today.

Botox

Botox is the brand name for a purified protein that is used to minimize the appearance of fine lines on the face. Botox works only on active wrinkles, which are wrinkles that are caused when you make facial expressions, such as smiling or frowning. When injected in small amounts, Botox weakens the muscles, reducing the facial movements that cause the wrinkles. The three areas most commonly treated with Botox are crow's feet, forehead lines, and frown lines between the eyes.

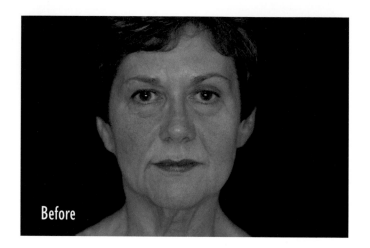

Before

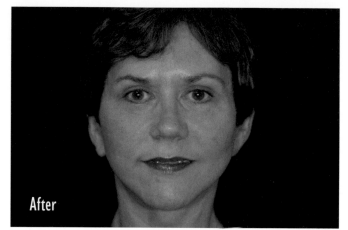

After

Facelift

Botox treatments take only about five to ten minutes in your plastic surgeon's office and don't require any form of anesthesia. A few injections are made into the area being treated using a tiny needle that causes only minimal, if any, discomfort. Typically, you can go back to your normal activities following Botox treatments. The effects of Botox treatments last about four to six months.

Following the injections, you'll be asked to avoid lying down or rubbing the treated area for several hours. This will help prevent the Botox from moving to other areas of your face. If the product does move, it can affect surrounding muscles, for instance, causing eyelids or brows to droop temporarily.

Microdermabrasion

For a skin refreshening technique that can repair fine lines and age spots without any downtime, consider microdermabrasion. This procedure, which may require a series of treatments to achieve the best results, involves the use of a very fine sandblaster to scrub off dead skin cells. The beauty of microdermabrasion is that you can get a treatment over the lunch hour and go right back to work. There's no pain, no swelling, and no lasting redness. As with most skin rejuvenation techniques, you'll need to avoid the sun and use sunscreen liberally after your treatment.

Wrinkle Fillers

Fillers are used to plump passive wrinkles, those lines and folds that are present even when you aren't making any facial expressions. These wrinkles are commonly due to things such as sun damage or smoking. Injectable fillers are commonly used to smooth nasolabial folds, smile lines, wrinkles around the lips, and forehead lines.

Fillers are popular because the procedure is quick and effective and doesn't involve any downtime. Results typically last from six to twelve months, but some types of fillers may last for several years. In general, the effects wear off more quickly in areas of the face that involve a lot of movement, such as the mouth and lips. You can expect more long-lasting results when treating areas that don't involve as much movement.

Different materials can be used as fillers. The most popular type of fillers is derived from hyaluronic acid, a substance found in all living organisms. This material is marketed under the brand names Restylane, Perlane, and Juvederm. When the substance is injected, it corrects lost volume in the skin, making wrinkles and lines less noticeable. Other materials used include hydroxy-appetite, sold under the name Radiesse. This material also is similar to a substance found in the human body. Usually injected into areas of the face that don't involve a lot of movement, it can provide long-lasting results. Polylactic acid, a material used to make sutures, is another injectable filler marketed under the brand name Sculptra.

Injections of this material stimulate the growth of collagen and may last several years. On the downside, it involves several months of repeated treatments before the effects can be seen.

Autologous fat transplanted from another area of the body, such as the abdomen or hips, is sometimes used as a wrinkle filler, but the results can be unpredictable. Finally, collagen injections used to be common but are rarely used anymore.

Laser Skin Resurfacing

Laser skin resurfacing can smooth fine lines, erase wrinkles, and minimize skin imperfections, such as broken blood vessels, age spots, and spider veins. It also can be used to remove excess facial hair. Lasers produce a beam of light that emits intense heat. This heat causes a controlled injury that eliminates the skin's imperfections. Doctors use two types of lasers to treat the skin: *ablative* and *non-ablative*. Ablative lasers, which are comparatively aggressive, remove an outer layer of skin and also may treat deeper tissues. Non-ablative lasers are less aggressive and focus only on tissues beneath the skin.

Carbon dioxide (CO_2) is considered the gold standard of laser skin resurfacing. The most aggressive of all lasers, it produces the most dramatic results, softening wrinkles and improving the appearance of sun-damaged skin. The CO_2 laser causes a controlled burn to the outer layer of skin and a heat injury to the deeper layer of tissue.

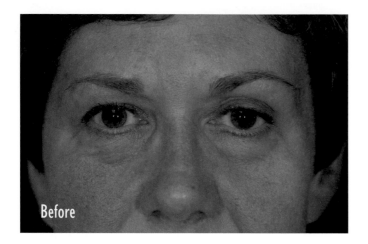

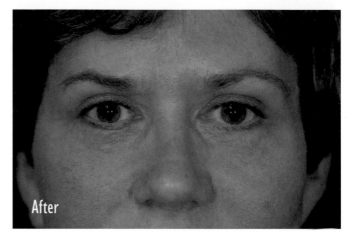

Upper and lower eyelid lifts

After your skin heals, it will appear softer, smoother, and firmer.

On the downside, this procedure poses the most risks and requires the longest recovery time. It is typically performed in a surgical suite and requires the use of anesthetics. You can expect your face to be very red and swollen for several weeks following your procedure. Redness can last from three to six months but can usually be covered by makeup. You'll need to wear dressings on your face for several days and may need to return to the doctor's office to change the dressings. Your physician also will give you detailed post-treatment instructions designed to promote healing and prevent infection.

Another ablative laser is the Erbium laser, which vaporizes the surface of the skin but doesn't cause any injury to the deeper tissues. Because of this, the results are usually not as remarkable as with the CO_2 laser, and deeper wrinkles usually don't show as much improvement. However, this method is considered safer than CO_2 laser resurfacing and involves a shorter healing period.

Fractional resurfacing is a newer method in which the laser targets only portions of the skin. This requires a series of about four to six treatments, and the results are similar to what can be achieved with the Erbium laser. The advantage of fractional resurfacing is that the skin heals in only two to three days, so you will see your results more quickly.

CHAPTER 12

Non-ablative devices use radio frequency waves to cause a heat injury to the deeper tissues beneath the skin. These types of treatments are ideal for treating fines lines and wrinkles and for general toning of the skin. Thermage is one of the most common devices for this, but other manufacturers also make devices that perform similar functions. Other lasers and intense pulsed light devices may be used to treat and eliminate broken blood vessels, brown age spots, spider veins, and unwanted hair. You may require a series of treatments to achieve the maximum effect.

These simple procedures take place in the doctor's office and may be performed by the doctor or by a trained technician. A topical anesthetic may be applied to the area being treated to minimize any discomfort. The entire procedure usually takes less than an hour and may take only fifteen minutes if you are only having a small area treated. There's no downtime associated with these types of laser procedures, and you can return immediately to your everyday activities.

Chemical Peels

A chemical peel involves the use of chemical solutions to remove the top layer of skin from your face. Once your skin heals, it appears softer and smoother. Chemical peels are commonly used to rejuvenate sun-damaged skin and can reduce the appearance of fine lines and other imperfections. Chemical peels are available in several strengths

Facelift and Neck Lift Facts

- Length of Surgery: 2 to 4 hours
- Type of Anesthesia: General, or local with sedation
- Hospital Stay: Optional overnight stay
- Pain Level: Mild
- Drains: Yes, usually removed the next day
- Compression Garment: Yes, neck support binder for at least 2 weeks
- Visible Sutures: Removed in 5 to 7 days in office; staples may remain for up to 2 weeks
- Activity Restrictions: No strenuous activity or heavy lifting for 6 weeks
- Return to Work: 1 to 3 weeks
- Final Outcome: 6 to 12 months

and types that result in superficial, medium depth, and deeper peels.

Light peels, which remove only the top layer of skin, are the most popular and require minimal or no recovery time. Medium peels remove the entire outer layer of skin to reduce or eliminate fine lines, surface wrinkles, and pigmentation problems. Complete healing takes three to five days with a medium peel. Deep peels use the strongest chemical solution of all the peels and produce the most dramatic results. However, complete healing from a deep peel may take seven to ten days, with progressive changes in the skin being seen for several months. Chemical peels are usually performed in the doctor's office, but deep peels may take place in a surgical suite. Light and medium peels typically take less than fifteen minutes, although deeper peels may take up to two hours. Anesthetics aren't required for any peels, but sedation may be used for deep peels to keep you relaxed and comfortable.

Any type of peel can cause redness, stinging, and irritation. With light peels, side effects are usually mild, and you can return immediately to your normal activities. Medium peels may cause discomfort and mild swelling that lasts about a week. Deep peels can cause severe swelling and redness. You may need someone to help you with your everyday routine for a few days after a deep peel, and you may have to wait a few weeks to return to your regular activities.

With light peels, you may want to repeat the procedure every three to four months to maintain your new look. The results of a medium peel may last about a year. And with deep peels, you can expect long-lasting results. Your plastic surgeon also will give you skin care advice to help you maintain your new fresh glow.

Thermal Skin Resurfacing

A newer treatment, known as *Portrait Plasma Skin Regeneration*, uses thermal energy to rejuvenate the skin. On the surface, it reduces the look of fine lines and deep wrinkles and improves discolored, sun-damaged skin; below the surface, the treatment stimulates growth of old, damaged collagen, thereby improving skin elasticity and texture.

There are four different kinds of treatment, and your doctor will choose one that is appropriate for your needs. To begin the procedure, a topical anesthetic is first applied to the skin, although the procedure is relatively painless. Then, as the doctor passes a hand-held device over the skin, plasma energy is released evenly across the skin. The device, however, never touches the skin.

In Closing

We hope this book has helped you gain a better understanding of bariatric plastic surgery and what it can do for you. In addition, we hope that you feel more comfortable about what to look for in a plastic surgeon and what to expect from the entire surgery process. If you're considering having any of the procedures described in this book, we encourage you to schedule a consultation with a board-certified plastic surgeon to discuss your options.

We can tell you from experience that the vast majority of our patients are extremely happy with the results of bariatric plastic surgery. For many patients, it gives them a sense that they have completed their journey both physically and psychologically. Reshaping your body with plastic surgery can open the door to a whole new life for you. It can give you a feeling of confidence you've never had before. And you may discover that you have a renewed zest for life and a desire to try new things and activities you never thought you could do.

Appendix A

Checklist of Questions to Ask Your Surgeon

It may be a good idea to take this checklist of questions with you to your consultation so you can refer to it during your discussion.

- ✓ Are you certified by the American Board of Plastic Surgery?

- ✓ Do you perform bariatric plastic surgery on a regular basis?

- ✓ May I see photographs of your previous work in bariatric patients?

- ✓ Which procedure or procedures do you recommend for me?

- ✓ Do you advise staging the procedures or combining them in a single operation?

- ✓ If you advise staging, how long will I have to wait before having my second surgery?

- ✓ If staging, how long will the entire process take before I see my final results?

- ✓ Where will you perform my surgery: hospital, surgery center, or office-based surgical suite?

- ✓ Is the facility accredited?

- ✓ What type of anesthesia will be used for my surgery and who will administer it?

- ✓ Will I be required to stay overnight in the hospital?

- ✓ Is there anything I can do to better prepare for surgery?

- ✓ What's involved in the recovery process?

- ✓ How long will it take to see my results?

- ✓ How long will it take to get back to my normal activities and to return to work?

✓ What are the side effects and risks associated with my procedure?

✓ How much pain should I expect to experience following surgery?

✓ What is the total cost for the surgery?

✓ Will insurance pay for any portion of my procedure?

✓ Do you offer any financing options?

✓ If I have complications, will I be financially responsible for the additional care required?

Appendix B

Body Mass Index Table																																			

	Normal						Overweight					Obese										Extreme Obesity														
BMI	19	20	21	22	23	24	25	26	27	28	29	30	31	32	33	34	35	36	37	38	39	40	41	42	43	44	45	46	47	48	49	50	51	52	53	54
Height (inches)											Body Weight (pounds)																									
58	91	96	100	105	110	115	119	124	129	134	138	143	148	153	158	162	167	172	177	181	186	191	196	201	205	210	215	220	224	229	234	239	244	248	253	258
59	94	99	104	109	114	119	124	128	133	138	143	148	153	158	163	168	173	178	183	188	193	198	203	208	212	217	222	227	232	237	242	247	252	257	262	267
60	97	102	107	112	118	123	128	133	138	143	148	153	158	163	168	174	179	184	189	194	199	204	209	215	220	225	230	235	240	245	250	255	261	266	271	276
61	100	106	111	116	122	127	132	137	143	148	153	158	164	169	174	180	185	190	195	201	206	211	217	222	227	232	238	243	248	254	259	264	269	275	280	285
62	104	109	115	120	126	131	136	142	147	153	158	164	169	175	180	186	191	196	202	207	213	218	224	229	235	240	246	251	256	262	267	273	278	284	289	295
63	107	113	118	124	130	135	141	146	152	158	163	169	175	180	186	191	197	203	208	214	220	225	231	237	242	248	254	259	265	270	278	282	287	293	299	304
64	110	116	122	128	134	140	145	151	157	163	169	174	180	186	192	197	204	209	215	221	227	232	238	244	250	256	262	267	273	279	285	291	296	302	308	314
65	114	120	126	132	138	144	150	156	162	168	174	180	186	192	198	204	210	216	222	228	234	240	246	252	258	264	270	276	282	288	294	300	306	312	318	324
66	118	124	130	136	142	148	155	161	167	173	179	186	192	198	204	210	216	223	229	235	241	247	253	260	266	272	278	284	291	297	303	309	315	322	328	334
67	121	127	134	140	146	153	159	166	172	178	185	191	198	204	211	217	223	230	236	242	249	255	261	268	274	280	287	293	299	306	312	319	325	331	338	344
68	125	131	138	144	151	158	164	171	177	184	190	197	203	210	216	223	230	236	243	249	256	262	269	276	282	289	295	302	308	315	322	328	335	341	348	354
69	128	135	142	149	155	162	169	176	182	189	196	203	209	216	223	230	236	243	250	257	263	270	277	284	291	297	304	311	318	324	331	338	345	351	358	365
70	132	139	146	153	160	167	174	181	188	195	202	209	216	222	229	236	243	250	257	264	271	278	285	292	299	306	313	320	327	334	341	348	355	362	369	376
71	136	143	150	157	165	172	179	186	193	200	208	215	222	229	236	243	250	257	265	272	279	286	293	301	308	315	322	329	338	343	351	358	365	372	379	386
72	140	147	154	162	169	177	184	191	199	206	213	221	228	235	242	250	258	265	272	279	287	294	302	309	316	324	331	338	346	353	361	368	375	383	390	397
73	144	151	159	166	174	182	189	197	204	212	219	227	235	242	250	257	265	272	280	288	295	302	310	318	325	333	340	348	355	363	371	378	386	393	401	408
74	148	155	163	171	179	186	194	202	210	218	225	233	241	249	256	264	272	280	287	295	303	311	319	326	334	342	350	358	365	373	381	389	396	404	412	420
75	152	160	168	176	184	192	200	208	216	224	232	240	248	256	264	272	279	287	295	303	311	319	327	335	343	351	359	367	375	383	391	399	407	415	423	431
76	156	164	172	180	189	197	205	213	221	230	238	246	254	263	271	279	287	295	304	312	320	328	336	344	353	361	369	377	385	394	402	410	418	426	435	443

Source: Adapted from *Clinical Guidelines on the Identification, Evaluation, and Treatment of Overweight and Obesity in Adults: The Evidence Report.*

Resources

American Board of Medical Specialties

1007 Church Street, Suite 404
Evanston, IL 60201-5913
Phone: 847-491-9091
Fax: 847-328-3596
www.abms.org

The American Board of Medical Specialties (ABMS), an organization of twenty-four approved medical specialty boards, oversees the board certification of physicians and surgeons. The ABMS Web site explains the criteria required to become board certified and offers a search feature to help you find board-certified physicians.

American Board of Plastic Surgery

Seven Penn Center
1635 Market Street
Suite 400
Philadelphia, PA 19103-2204

Phone: 215-587-9322
Fax: 215-587-9622
www.abplsurg.org

The American Board of Plastic Surgery (ABPS) promotes safe and ethical plastic surgery for the public by setting high standards for the education, examination, and certification of plastic surgeons. On the ABPS Web site, you can find FAQs that explain the board certification process.

American Society for Bariatric Surgery

100 SW 75th St.
Suite 201
Gainesville, FL 32607
Phone: 352-331-4900
Fax: 352-331-4975
www.asbs.org

This group of bariatric surgeons aims to advance the medical specialty of bariatric surgery. The organization's Web site includes a "patients" section where you can find information about bariatric surgery options, a BMI calculator, and a physician finder that lets you search for a bariatric surgeon in your area.

The American Society of Bariatric Plastic Surgeons

1540 South Coast Highway, Suite 203
Laguna Beach, CA 92651
Phone: 800-946-9512
www.asbps.org

Established by plastic surgeons that specialize in body contouring surgery for patients who have lost significant amounts of weight, the ASBP's goals is to help patients find knowledgeable and experienced plastic surgeons. Its members are certified by the American Board of Plastic Surgeons and most are members of the American Society of Plastic Surgeons as well as the American Society of Aesthetic Plastic Surgery or the Canadian Society of Plastic Surgeons. Along with the "Find a Surgeon" feature, the Web site also features information on procedures, articles about plastic surgery, and links to other helpful information.

American Society of Aesthetic Plastic Surgery

11081 Winners Circle
Los Alamitos, CA 90720-2813
Phone: 888-ASAPS-11 (888-272-7711)
(physician referrals)
www.surgery.org

Founded in 1967, ASAPS is a professional organization of board-certified plastic surgeons who specialize in aesthetic plastic surgery. The organization has 2,100 members in the United States, Canada, and many other countries. The Web site features a "consumers" section where you can view details—including average prices—of numerous procedures, including several bariatric plastic surgery procedures. Tips on how to choose a surgeon and a "Find-a-Surgeon" feature also arc available.

American Society of Plastic Surgeons

444 East Algonquin Road
Arlington Heights, IL 60005
Phone: 847-228-9900; 888-4-PLASTIC
888-475-2784 (physician referrals)
www.plasticsurgery.org

Established in 1931, the American Society of Plastic Surgeons (ASPS) is the world's largest plastic surgery specialty organization. Composed of board-certified plastic surgeons who perform cosmetic and reconstructive plastic surgery, the ASPS encourages high standards of training, ethics, physician practice, and research in plastic surgery. On the "patients & consumers" section of the society's Web site, you'll find detailed information on a variety of procedures, photo galleries, tips on planning your surgery, and more.

Obesity Action Coalition

4511 North Himes Avenue
Suite 250
Tampa, FL 33614
Phone: 800-717-3117
www.obesityaction.org

Educating patients, their families, and the public is one of the main goals of the Obesity Action Coalition (OAC). The OAC also aims to improve access to medical treatments for obese patients and advocates for safe and effective treatments for obese individuals. On the organization's Web site, you can find an online BMI calculator as well as patient stories and a forum where people can share their experiences.

ObesityHelp, Inc.

8001 Irvine Center Drive
Suite 1270
Irvine, CA 92618
Phone: 1-866-WLS-INFO (866-957-4636)
www.obesityhelp.com

Established in 1998 as a peer support community for the morbidly obese, ObesityHelp is dedicated to providing education and support to individuals affected by obesity. On the ObesityHelp Web site, you'll find a wealth of information on bariatric surgery as well as on plastic surgery after weight loss. You also can log on to chat rooms and online forums where people discuss their own experiences with bariatric plastic surgery.

Obesity Society

8630 Fenton Street
Suite 814
Silver Spring, MD 20910
Phone: 301-563-6526
www.obesity.org

Established in 1982, the Obesity Society encourages research on the causes, prevention, and treatment of obesity. The organization also publishes *Obesity,* the leading journal in the field. The Web site offers a wealth of information on research, treatment, prevention, discrimination, and additional topics related to obesity.

U.S. National Library of Medicine

8600 Rockville Pike
Bethesda, MD 20894
www.nlm.nih.gov
www.nlm.nih.gov/medlineplus

MedlinePlus is a service of the U.S. National Library of Medicine and the National Institutes of Health. The consumer-oriented Web site includes authoritative information on more than 650 health-related topics. You also can view videos of surgical procedures and take advantage of more than 165 interactive tutorials on a variety of health topics.

Glossary

abdominoplasty: the medical term for a tummy tuck

ablative: a type of laser that removes or destroys the outer layer of the skin

advance health-care directive: a legal document that details your wishes for health-care should you be unable to communicate those wishes

allium cepa: an onion extract that is used in some products to minimize the appearance of scars

anchor breast lift: see *Wise pattern breast lift*

anesthesia: any one of a number of agents used during surgery to block pain and induce drowsiness or a deep sleep in a patient

areola: the shaded area surrounding the nipple

arm lift: a surgical procedure in which excess skin and fatty deposits are removed from the upper arms

aspirate: a technique that employs suction to withdraw fluids from the body, usually through a needle

belt lipectomy: another term used for a *lower body lift*

blepharoplasty: upper and lower eyelid surgery

body lift: see *lower body lift*

brachioplasty: the medical term for an *arm lift*

breast augmentation: a surgical procedure that increases the size of the breasts by inserting implants; see also *breast implant*

breast implant: a sac with an outer shell made of a silicone rubberlike substance that is filled with either sterile saline or silicone gel

breast lift: a surgical procedure that lifts and reshapes saggy breasts

browlift: a surgical procedure used to minimize a drooping brow

buttock autoaugmentation: a surgical procedure in which your own tissue is used to add projection to your buttocks

cannula: a long, thin tube used to suction fat during liposuction

capsular contracture: a complication following breast augmentation in which scar tissue contracts and squeezes the implant

central body lift: another term used for a *lower body lift*

cervicoplasty: the medical term for a *neck lift*

circumferential torsoplasty: another term used for a *lower body lift*

crescent breast lift: a type of breast lift that involves a crescent-shaped incision on the areola

deep venous thrombosis (DVT): a blood clot, usually in the leg

dog ear: a complication in which tissue bunches or bulges at the extremity of a scar

diastasis: a medical condition in which the vertical muscles of the abdominal wall separate

doughnut breast lift: a type of breast lift in which a circular incision is made around the areola

elastomer: a rubberlike substance used in the outer shell of breast implants

electrocardiogram (EKG or ECG): a procedure used to diagnose abnormalities in heartbeat

electrocautery: a method in which a small electric current is used during surgery to cauterize tissue

epinephrine: a drug used during surgery to constrict blood vessels and to prolong the effects of local anesthetics

extended brachioplasty: a type of arm lift in which the incisions extend beyond the elbow or beyond the underarm to the side of the chest

extended SMAS facelift: a type of facelift that minimizes lines around the nose and mouth

extended tummy tuck: a type of tummy tuck in which the incisions extend beyond the hip bones

fascia: connective tissues that cover the muscles of the abdominal wall

fascial plication: a surgical procedure in which the fascia is tightened using sutures

flanks: the fleshy part of the body between the ribs and the hip

forehead lift: see *browlift*

free nipple graft: a method used for breast reduction surgery in which the nipple is completely detached from the breast and then reattached

gynecomastia: a medical condition in which the male breasts enlarge

hematoma: a collection of blood within the tissue of the body

hernia: a condition in which an internal organ or tissue bulges through weakened tissues, usually on the abdomen

hyaluronic acid: a filler material injected in the skin to soften the appearance of lines and wrinkles

hypertrophic scars: thick, raised scars caused by excessive tissue growth at the site of an incision

incentive spirometer: a device used to encourage deep breathing following a surgical procedure

inframammary fold: the crease or fold beneath the breast

inner thigh lift: a surgical procedure in which excess skin and fat is removed from the inner thighs

inverted T breast lift: see *Wise pattern breast lift*

keloid: a thick, raised, uneven scar caused by excessive tissue growth at the site of a surgical incision or wound

labia: the lips of the vagina

laparoscopically: a surgical technique in which a small camera is inserted into the surgical area through very tiny incisions

liposuction: the surgical removal of localized fat deposits in the body by using suction through a small cannula

lollipop breast lift: see *vertical breast lift*

lower body lift: a surgical procedure in which an incision is made around the torso to remove excess skin and fat from the abdomen, hips, and back

lymphatic system: part of the circulatory system

mammogram: a procedure using x-ray technology to detect cancer in the breasts

mastopexy: the medical term for a *breast lift*

medial thighplasty: the medical term for an *inner thigh lift*

monitored anesthesia care (MAC): a technique for administering anesthesia while continuously monitoring a patient's vital signs

monsplasty: the medical term for a *pubic lift*

mons pubis: the medical term for the pubic area

nasolabial folds: the lines that extend from the sides of the nose toward the corners of the mouth

necrosis: tissue death

nipple/areola complex: the nipple and surrounding shaded area

non-ablative: a type of laser that treats tissues beneath the skin but does not remove the outer layer of skin

opioid: narcotic medication

pain pump: another term for a *pain relief ball*

pain relief ball: a catheter inserted into a surgical site that delivers local anesthetics to provide post-surgical pain relief

panniculectomy: a surgical procedure to remove a *panniculus*

panniculus: a large apron of skin that hangs in folds from the abdomen

patient-controlled analgesia (PCA): a method used to allow a patient to administer pre-measured doses of pain medication

pectoral muscle: the muscle located between the breasts and the ribs

platysmaplasty: a surgical procedure that tightens the muscles within the neck

polylactic acid: a filler material used to smooth facial lines and wrinkles

post-operative anesthesia care unit (PACU): the area where patients are taken immediately following surgery

ptosis: the medical term for sagging breasts

pubic lift: a surgical procedure that restores the contours of the pubic area; see *monsplasty*

pulmonary embolism: a life-threatening condition in which a blood clot lodges in the lung

rhytidectomy: the medical term for a facelift

sedation: a type of anesthesia in which sedatives are administered to the patient to induce drowsiness or unconsciousness as a way to eliminate pain during a surgical procedure

seroma: a collection of clear fluid within the body

short-scar brachioplasty: a type of arm lift in which the incision is usually restricted to the upper one-third of the upper arm

silicone: a rubberlike substance used in the outer shell of breast implants

silicone gel: a gelatinous substance made of *silicone* that is sometimes used to fill *breast implants*

sleep apnea: a medical condition in which a person stops breathing for periods of time while sleeping

SMAS facelift: a type of facelift that tightens the layer of facial muscle beneath the skin in addition to tightening the skin

standard brachioplasty: a type of arm lift that usually extends from the elbow to the underarm

Steri-Strips: a type of surgical tape that can be used on the surface of the skin to keep incisions closed

subcutaneous: below the skin

subcutaneous musculoaponeurotic system (SMAS): the layer of muscle beneath the skin on the face

subglandular: the placement of a *breast implant* beneath the breast tissue but above the pectoral muscle

submuscular: the placement of a *breast implant* partially below the pectoral muscle

thighplasty: the medical term for a thigh lift

tummy tuck: a surgical procedure in which excess skin and fat are permanently removed from the abdomen and in which muscles of the abdominal wall may be tightened

umbilicus: the medical term for the navel

undermining: a surgical technique used to separate skin from underlying tissues

upper body lift: a surgical procedure in which excess skin and fat are permanently removed from the breasts, male chest, and back

vertical breast lift: a type of breast lift involving a vertical incision from the areola to the inframammary fold and a circular incision around the areola

Wise pattern breast lift: a breast lift that involves three incisions—a horizontal incision along the inframammary fold, a vertical incision from the areola to the inframammary fold, and a circular incision around the areola; also referred to as an *anchor breast lift* or *inverted T breast lift*

Index

compression hose, 55
compression sleeves, 43
compression stockings, 93
computed axial tomography (CAT or CT scan), 64
connective tissue disorders, 8, 101
conscious sedation, 42
consent forms, 38
constipation, 32, 53, 54
consultation with plastic surgeon, 19–27
    expectations, 19, 20
    preparation, 20
continuing medical education, 14
core body temperature, 43
costs, 25–27
Coumadin, 33
credit application, 26
crescent breast lift, 99
crow's feet, 135

D

death of fat tissue, 79
deep breathing instructions, 48, 52, 66, 86
deep skin peels, 139
deep structures, 51
    injuries to, 51
deep vein thrombosis (DVT), 43, 51, 93
delayed healing, 50, 78, 93
Demerol, 53
depression, 49
diabetes, 8
diastasis, 58
Dilaudid, 53
dizziness, 54
dog ear scar, 69
doughnut breast lift, 99
drains
    see surgical drains
driving, 56
drooping brow, 130

drowsiness, 53
dry mouth, 47
durable power of attorney for health care, 36

E

Eklund mammogram technique, 113
elective cosmetic surgery, 26
electrocardiogram (EKG or ECG), 30
electrocautery, 37, 44
epidural anesthesia, 41
epinephrine, 43, 44
Erbium laser, 138
expectations, 5, 7, 19, 20
extended abdominoplasty, 60
extended brachioplasty, 117
extended SMAS facelift, 130
extended tummy tuck, 59

F

face and neck procedures, 129–140
    chronic pain, 135
    hair loss, 135
    numbness, 135
    pain management, 132, 134
    recovery, 132, 134
    risk factors, 134, 135
facelift, 4, 129, 130
facial swelling, 132
failed treatments, 26
fascia, 58
    repair, 61, 69
fascial plication, 61
fasting, 36, 39
fat cells, 44
fat deposits, 79, 115, 131
    removal with liposuction, 44, 59
fat grafts, 131
fat injections, 72, 73, 76, 83
fat necrosis, 79, 93

fecal contamination, 77, 78
Federation of State Medical Boards, 14
fees, 25–27
fellowship, 14
financial planning, 27
financing options, 19, 26, 27
    credit application, 26
fluid buildup, 45, 93
fluid drainage, 46, 74, 93
    see also surgical drains
fluid intake, 55
Foley catheter, 43
follow-up appointments, 20, 57, 93
Food and Drug Administration (FDA), 101
forehead lift, 130
forehead lines, 135, 137
forehead numbness, 132
former patients, 23, 24
fractional face resurfacing, 138
free nipple graft, 107, 108
    disadvantages, 108
free nipple transfer, 108
frown lines, 135, 137

G

gauze dressings, 62, 63, 74, 85, 110, 115, 126
general anesthesia, 40, 41
glandular breast tissue, 106, 114, 115
goals, 7, 19, 20, 23
good candidates for bariatric plastic surgery, 4–8,
  21

H

hair loss, 135
hair removal, 139
headaches, 26
healing problems, 8, 30
    smoking, 8
healing tips, 56

health care decisions, 36
health care declaration, 36
health care financing lenders, 27
health care legal documents, 36
heart disease, 5, 8, 21
heart monitor, 40
heart rate, 47
heart tissues
    damage to, 30
heartburn, 54
heat loss prevention, 42, 43
heating pads, 55
heavy eyelids, 130
hemoglobin, 29
hemophilia, 30
hematoma, 49
    with breast augmentation procedures, 112
    drainage, 49
    with facelift, 134
    severe, 50
herbal supplements, 21, 33
    to avoid before surgery, 33
hernias, 22, 26, 64, 65
    repair, 26, 64, 65
high blood pressure, 21
high-lateral-tension tummy tuck, 60
home aide, 34
home health care organizations, 34
hospital training, 13
hydrocodone, 32
hydromorphone, 53
hyluronic acid, 137
hypertension, 5, 8
hypertrophic scars, 50

I

ibuprofen, 33, 53
ice packs, 55
immune system, 9, 52

recovery, 127
    risk factors, 128
upper torsoplasty, 122
urinalysis, 29
urinary catheters, 43, 76, 86
urine test, 29

V

vertical breast lift, 98, 99
vertical incision breast reduction, 107
Vicodin, 32, 53
vital signs, 39, 46
vitamin B-12, 32
vitamin C, 32
vitamin E, 33, 57
vitamins, 21, 29, 32
    to avoid before surgery, 33
vomiting, 9, 21, 36, 53

W

walking, 55, 76, 87
    after surgery, 47, 48, 52, 66, 93
walking difficulties
    due to panniculus, 26
warming pads or blankets, 43
weight fluctuations, 70, 96
weight loss support group, 24
white blood cell count, 29
Wise pattern breast lift, 98, 125
wound care, 66, 76
wound healing, 8, 9, 33, 45
    problems, 50
wound separation, 78, 93
wound therapy treatment, 50
wrinkle fillers, 137

X

X-ray, 30

About the Authors

Every patient is beautiful and unique. I believe that cosmetic surgery can renew and accentuate one's outer beauty, while enhancing inner beauty and a higher sense of self-confidence.

—Thomas B. McNemar, M.D., F.A.C.S.

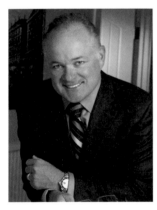

Thomas B. McNemar, M.D., F.A.C.S., is a plastic surgeon in private practice with offices in Tracy and San Ramon, California. He attended the Medical College of Ohio, where he made the decision to pursue a surgical career. After completing a general surgery residency at the Cleveland Clinic, he continued his surgical education at Akron City Hospital as a plastic surgery fellow. He rounded out his formal education at the Bunke Clinic in San Francisco, California, as an attending fellow specializing in hand and microvascular surgery. Dr. McNemar has been recognized as a leader in treating post-bariatric surgery patients, and he has lectured extensively on the subject. He is also co-author of *Your Complete Guide to Breast Augmentation and Body Contouring* (Addicus Books 2006). Dr. McNemar is married and the father of two children. He and his family enjoy the outdoor leisure ac tivities and fine-art opportunities the Bay area has to offer. He enjoys skiing, bicycling, and the culinary arts. Dr. McNemar can be reached through his Web site:

www.bariatricplasticsurgeon.com

Many patients who have had dramatic weight losses see the excess skin as a reminder of their former self—when they were overweight. As a plastic surgeon, I have the opportunity to help them overcome this psychological hurdle in their weight loss journey.

—John LoMonaco, M.D., F.A.C.S.

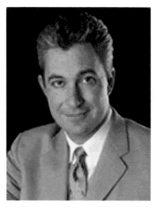 **John LoMonaco, M.D., F.A.C.S.,** attended Medical School at the University of Texas Health Science Center at Houston and completed his nine years of postgraduate training there as well. He trained at major hospitals in the Texas Medical Center, including Memorial-Hermann Hospital and M.D. Anderson Cancer Institute. During his training, he conducted laboratory research for two years at the Medical School studying tissue healing and helping develop skin substitutes for burn victims.

Dr. LoMonaco graduated from a rigorous residency in general surgery and received board certification by the American Board of Surgery. He then went on to complete an accredited fellowship in plastic surgery and received board certification in plastic surgery during his first year of practice. During his formal training, Dr. LoMonaco participated in more than 5,000 surgical procedures.

After graduation, Dr. LoMonaco taught plastic surgery for two years at the University of Texas Health Science Center at Houston and served as Director of Plastic Surgery at the LBJ Hospital. In 1999, he traveled to El Salvador as part of a medical relief mission to perform surgery on children with facial deformities.

Dr. LoMonaco's interests include all aspects of plastic surgery, with a special interest in breast and body contouring surgery. His office is near the Texas Medical Center and is equipped with its own operating facility. He also maintains operating privileges at several Medical Center hospitals and is a member of both local and national medical societies. Dr. LoMonaco can be reached through his Web site:

www.drlomonaco.com

About the Authors

My profession is one in which you build lifelong relationships with patients, and that's very important to me. It's so rewarding to use my skills and abilities to help my patients feel better about their appearance, and in many cases, improve the quality of their lives.

—Mitchel D. Krieger, M.D., F.A.C.S.

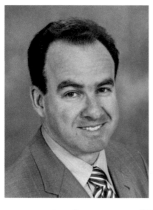

Mitchel D. Krieger, M.D., F.A.C.S., is a plastic surgeon, specializing in aesthetic and reconstructive surgery, in Fairfax, Virginia. He attended medical school at Albany Medical College, completing its accelerated six-year biomedical program with Rensselaer Polytechnic Institute.

A former military surgeon, Dr. Krieger completed surgical training in San Francisco and Washington, D.C. He served as a consultant surgeon to the British military during the first Gulf War and later served on the teaching faculty at the Medical College of Georgia, helping to train plastic surgeons residents. Leaving military service in 1997, he entered private practice in Northern Virginia. He brings nearly twenty years worth of experience as both a general surgeon and as a plastic surgeon in treating bariatric patients. Dr. Krieger is double board-certified in general surgery and plastic surgery. He is a Member of the American Society of Plastic Surgeons and the American Society of Bariatric Plastic Surgeons, and he is a Fellow of the American College of Surgeons and the American Society for Laser Medicine and Surgery.

Acknowledged by many as one of the most experienced bariatric plastic surgeons in the country, he is constantly striving to improve the overall patient experience. Providing cosmetic surgery options to patients who have recently undergone bariatric procedures, he is able to help people more fully enjoy their new, slimmed-down bodies. His involvement with the Bariatric Center of Excellent at Inova Fair Oaks Hospital has given Dr. Krieger a unique ability to help optimize patient's surgical results. Adroit in a wide array of procedures, Dr. Krieger readily consults with patients to bring them the latest techniques suitable to their needs and desires.

Dr. Krieger enjoys travel to far-off destinations but enjoys his downtime closer to home by fishing and exploring the Chesapeake Bay. A longtime oenophile, Dr. Krieger has received extensive training in wine education and will soon complete certification as a sommelier. Dr. Krieger can be reached through his Web site:
www.virginiaplasticsurgery.com

Consumer Health Titles from Addicus Books

Visit our online catalog at www.AddicusBooks.com

After Mastectomy—
Healing Physically and Emotionally $14.95

Bariatric Plastic Surgery $24.95

Cancers of the Mouth and Throat—
A Patient's Guide to Treatment $14.95

Cataracts—A Patient's Guide to Treatment . . . $14.95

Colon & Rectal Cancer—
A Patient's Guide to Treatment $14.95

Coping with Psoriasis—
A Patient's Guide to Treatment $14.95

Coronary Heart Disease—
A Guide to Diagnosis and Treatment $15.95

Countdown to Baby. $14.95

The Courtin Concept—Six Keys to Great
Skin at Any Age $19.95

Elder Care Made Easier $16.95

Exercising through Your Pregnancy $17.95

The Fertility Handbook—
A Guide to Getting Pregnant $14.95

The Healing Touch—Keeping the Doctor/Patient
Relationship Alive under Managed Care . . . $9.95

LASIK—A Guide to Laser Vision Correction . . $14.95

Living with P.C.O.S.—
Polycystic Ovarian Syndrome $14.95

Look Out Cancer Here I Come $19.95

Lung Cancer—
A Guide to Treatment & Diagnosis $14.95

The Macular Degeneration Source Book $14.95

The New Fibromyalgia Remedy $19.95

The Non-Surgical Facelift Book—
A Guide to Facial Rejuvenation Procedures . $14.95

Overcoming Metabolic Syndrome $14.95

Overcoming Postpartum
Depression and Anxiety $14.95

Overcoming Prescription Drug Addiction . . . $19.95

Overcoming Urinary Incontinence $19.95

A Patient's Guide to Dental Implants. $14.95

Prostate Cancer—
A Patient's Guide to Treatment $14.95

Simple Changes—The Boomer's Guide
to a Healthier, Happier Life $9.95

A Simple Guide to Thyroid Disorders $14.95

Straight Talk about Breast Cancer—
From Diagnosis to Recovery $15.95

The Stroke Recovery Book—
A Guide for Patients and Families $14.95

The Surgery Handbook—A Guide
to Understanding Your Operation $14.95

Understanding Lumpectomy—
A Treatment Guide for Breast Cancer $14.95

Understanding Parkinson's Disease—
A Self-Help Guide $14.95

Understanding Peyronie's Disease $16.95

Understanding Your Living Will $12.95

Your Complete Guide to Breast Augmentation
& Body Contouring $21.95

Your Complete Guide to Breast Reduction
& Breast Lifts $21.95

Your Complete Guide to Facial Cosmetic Surgery
. . . . $19.95

Your Complete Guide to Facelifts $21.95

Your Complete Guide to Nose Reshaping . . . $21.95

To Order Books:

Visit us online at: www.addicusbooks.com

Call toll free: 800-352-2873

For discounts on bulk purchases,
call our Special Sales Dept. at
(402) 330-7493

Please send:

_____copies of _____
(Title of book)

at $_____each   TOTAL: _____

Nebraska residents add 5% sales tax   _____

Shipping/Handling

    $5.00 postage for first book.   _____

    $1.20 postage for each additional book   _____

TOTAL ENCLOSED: _____

Name _____

Address _____

City _____State_____Zip _____

    ☐ **Visa**   ☐ **MasterCard**   ☐ **American Express**

Credit card number _____Expiration date _____

Order by credit card, personal check or money order. Send to:

Addicus Books
Mail Order Dept.
P.O. Box 45327
Omaha, NE 68145
Or, order **TOLL FREE: 800-352-2873**
or online at
www.AddicusBooks.com